HEALTH CARE ROULETTE

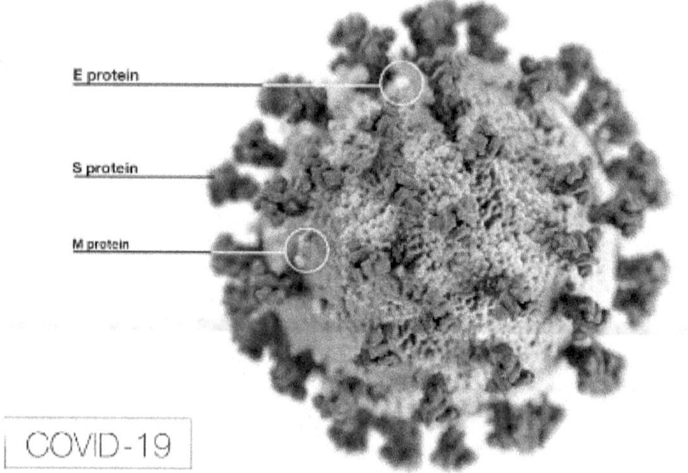

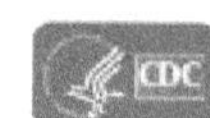

Adulterated and misbranded foreign drugs are infiltrating your medicine cabinet. The coronavirus is making your medications unavailable. Pharmacy benefit managers are rendering your medications unaffordable.

HEALTH CARE ROULETTE

What's in Your Prescription Bottle?

By Randolph George Tammara, PharmD, CDE, MPH

ISBN-13: 9798649452892

This book is dedicated to one very special pharmacist, my father, Steve Tammara, as well as the generations of community pharmacists in Philadelphia and beyond who, since colonial times, have provided their patients with unparalleled personal, professional, and clinical services. I cannot begin to count how many times I witnessed my father go above and beyond the call of duty, not only for his patients but also for people he did not even know. Just as George Bailey, the protagonist of Frank Capra's 1945 *It's a Wonderful Life*, never left a family without a roof over its head, Steve Tammara never left a sick patient without his or her medication, regardless of the patient's ability to pay.

I owe a debt of gratitude for the education that I received at Temple University School of Pharmacy.

The MPH program at Arcadia University became the missing piece of the puzzle that I needed to finally complete my work on *Health Care Roulette*. My capstone paper and presentation, "The Relationship between Not Taking Medication as Prescribed in the Last 12 Months Due to Cost among Patients with Diabetes Taking Insulin," was the culmination of decades of health-related observations and interactions in the pharmacy and in the classroom, as both a student and a teacher. Despite all the scientific advances we have accomplished in medicine and technology, disparities in access to health care are still prevalent, and vulnerable populations continue to be marginalized.

This book serves as a giant thank-you to Big Pharma and the Food and Drug Administration (FDA). As this book goes to print, Big Pharma is racing to find treatments, cures, and vaccines to combat the deadly COVID-19 pandemic. Without the innovations provided by the research and development of Big Pharma, we would have little hope of conquering COVID-19. FDA protects our food and pharmaceutical supply chain from being breached by deadly contaminants and impurities. FDA is our guardian angel, the gatekeeper, providing a safety net that filters out adulterated, misbranded, and outright counterfeit prescription drugs before they reach our medicine cabinets. Without FDA in our corner, we would all be dropping dead from adulterated and misbranded counterfeit drugs.

Unfortunately, FDA has limited authority beyond the United States. With the majority of pharmaceutical ingredients originating from sketchy overseas sources, FDA has seen its protective cloak circumvented by unscrupulous profiteers who are manufacturing substandard and deadly medications and introducing them into the global pharmaceutical supply chain.

Finally, this book recognizes a very special set of caregivers: direct support professionals (DSPs), who provide care for a multitude of physically and intellectually disabled individuals, many of whom are casualties of the diabetes epidemic that we are experiencing. As a pharmacist with a nearly thirty-year career and a certified diabetes educator, it has been my privilege to have worked with and trained hundreds of DSP caregivers in diabetes. This public health approach, using the "train the trainer" model, has allowed for exponential dissemination of knowledge as these DSP caregivers engage in primary, secondary, and tertiary prevention of diabetes in their individuals (residents/patients), their individuals' families, and themselves. Furthermore, caregivers and individuals in the mental health community have been my inspiration to further my education so that I can continue to make a difference in the lives of these populations; both have had a profound impact on my personal and professional paths in life.

The DSPs with whom I have crossed paths over the decades are the most patient, caring, and compassionate people I have ever encountered. Living under the same roof as their individuals and assisting them with activities of daily living, DSPs treat their individuals as if they are family members. DSPs assist those with disabilities in achieving self-directed lives and contributing to the communities in which they live.

TABLE OF CONTENTS

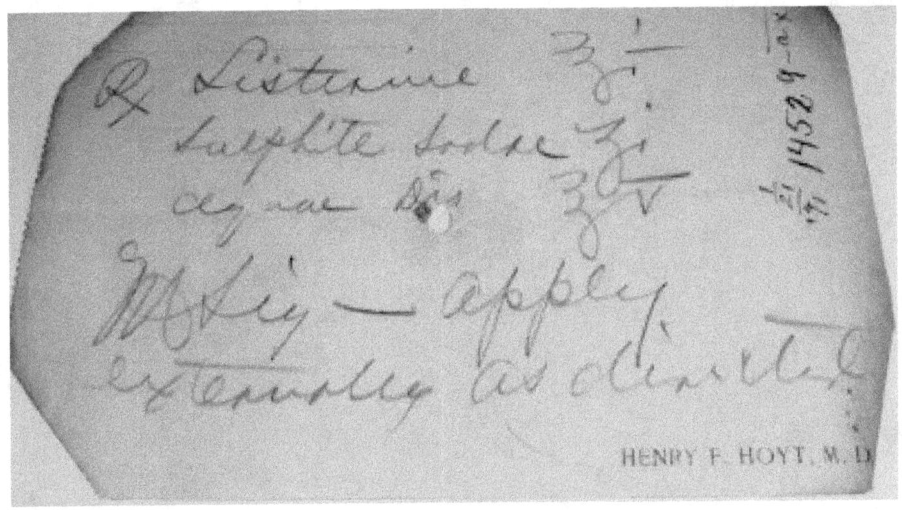

AUTHOR'S NOTE

Since the inception of community pharmacy over two hundred years ago, most small community pharmacists have refused to turn away a patient, even people who could not afford their prescriptions. If an indigent patient had no money, the charge was either waived or paid out over a few weeks or months, with no questions asked. Equally as important, the medications were manufactured in the United States under the protective cloak of the Food and Drug Administration (FDA).

State-administered Medicaid plans rightfully mandate that patients who cannot afford their prescription co-pays must still receive their lifesaving medications. But privately run Medicare, government, and commercial plans are often administered by for-profit pharmacy benefit managers (PBMs). PBMs, by manipulating restrictive drug formularies, prior authorizations, and unaffordable co-pays, redirect prescribing habits toward those medications that are most profitable for the PBMs themselves, rather than what the physician originally considered therapeutically best for the patient. Furthermore, these robber barons force pharmacists (by inflicting harsh penalties upon them) to turn away asthma patients who cannot afford their lifesaving inhalers, diabetic patients who cannot afford their life-sustaining insulin, and HIV patients who can develop resistance and die if they miss even one dose of their antiviral medications. Even if a compassionate pharmacist wants to help a needy patient by waiving a co-pay on a lifesaving drug, and even if the patient will otherwise die, PBMs contractually prohibit the pharmacist from intervening. In a recent study, medication adherence was compared among 34,475 patients with type 2 diabetes. Higher medication co-payment amounts were associated with lower patient medication adherence. Additionally, fixed co-pay plans were associated with higher persistence compared to three-tier plans (Henk, 2018). These unaffordable co-payments correlate with the high rates of morbidity and mortality that diabetes patients are forced to endure (Cefalu et al., 2018). Austvoll-Dahlgren et al. (2008) identified policies that aim to shift the financial burden from insurers to patients, often resulting in patients foregoing their lifesaving medications due to unaffordability. A quick Google search yields innumerable anecdotal references that prove PBMs are to blame for the negative health outcomes that result from medication nonadherence. Medication adherence or nonadherence is the phenomenon of patients taking their medication as prescribed versus foregoing their life-sustaining medications for some reason—in this case, the unaffordability of their co-payments.

Here is a clip from the popular television series *New Amsterdam* that addresses the life or death financial hardships being faced by persons with diabetes:

https://www.newsbusters.org/blogs/culture/julia-seymour/2019/09/25/
new-amsterdam-attacks-pharma-extortionists-season-2-premiere

Gourzoulidis et al. (2017) reviewed thirty-eight studies that examined the relationship between co-pays, medication adherence, and outcomes in both diabetes and heart failure. The results indicated that increased adherence correlates with positive health outcomes in both diabetes and heart failure. This review also found that higher co-pays may result in poor health and economic outcomes. Lower co-pays were associated with higher medication adherence in patients with diabetes and heart failure, demonstrating an inverse relationship between co-pays and adherence. Equal in significance to the formal scientific studies are the numerous and continuous anecdotal reports of people dying due to insulin nonadherence. This financially induced suffering is going unheeded by profiteering insurance companies, PBMs, and regulatory bodies. Cefalu et al. (2018) have established that working-class people, as well as senior citizens on fixed incomes, often have to choose between putting food on the table and taking their life-sustaining medications. The scientific literature has already shown the connection between medication co-pays and adherence (Gourzoulidis et al., 2017; Lyles et al., 2016; Pawasakar et al., 2018; Shah, 2009; Tamblyn et al., 2001). As mentioned, Gourzoulidis et al. have established the association between adherence and health outcomes. For example, in a sampling of the studies that were reviewed by these researchers, an increase in co-pay of ten dollars resulted in a 6 percent decrease in adherence; an increase in the co-pay of twenty dollars resulted in a 25 percent decrease in adherence. Medication nonadherence directly correlates with negative health outcomes (Cefalu et al., 2018; Ember, 2019). Increased cost sharing for prescription drugs in elderly persons and welfare recipients was followed by reductions in use of essential drugs and a higher rate of serious adverse events and emergency department visits associated with these reductions in medication usage (Tamblyn et al., 2001).

Hence it is already documented in the literature that co-pays affect adherence, and it is already documented in the literature that adherence affects health outcomes. *When people cannot afford their medications, they will not take their medications, and they will suffer physical complications and early death as a result of not taking their medications.* Shah (2009) identified a positive correlation between first-fill adherence of diabetes prescriptions and hemoglobin A1C. Hemoglobin A1C is a clinical parameter that is used diagnostically and is also the gold standard in assessing the health status of individuals with diabetes (American Diabetes Association [ADA], 2018).

As a second-generation pharmacist, certified diabetes educator, and an advocate for public health, I cannot morally deny a diabetes patient his or her lifesaving insulin simply because he or she cannot afford the co-pay. As such, I have chosen to pursue a career in public health and long-term care consulting rather than having to watch patients literally cry at the pharmacy counter when they are informed of their unaffordable insulin co-pays. Below is a link to an article about a woman who had to admit herself to the emergency room to get insulin, just for survival. The article goes on to describe the online black market for insulin, where patients are forced to purchase discounted insulin from anonymous sources, risking their lives just to try and stay alive. Despite the uncertainty of the origin and purity of products purchased on the black market, type 1 diabetics are forced to roll the dice because they will quickly fall into the deadly condition of diabetic ketoacidosis (DKA) if they do not take their insulin as prescribed on a daily basis. There is a direct correlation between not taking medication as prescribed (including insulin) due to cost and adverse health outcomes. Viral infections, including COVID-19, place diabetics at a higher risk of DKA, dehydration, and electrolyte imbalances. Sepsis and shock are some of the more serious complications that some people with COVID-19 have experienced. If the blood sugar of a person with diabetes registers high (greater than 240 mg/dl) more than two times in a row, the American Diabetes Association (ADA) recommends checking for ketones to avoid DKA. Contact your physician or call 911 immediately if you suspect you are in need of medical attention for DKA or any other medical condition. If you cannot afford your insulin, the ADA website recommends visiting InsulinHelp.org to find resources (ADA, 2018).

https://www.wptv.com/news/national/when-diabetics-cant-afford-insulin-they-turn-to-the-black-market-this-michigan-woman-helps-them-do-it

Here is another example of how diabetic patients are dying because they can no longer afford the insulin that was originally given to the world for free. The reader is encouraged *not* to take the author's word but rather to simply scan the QR code with a cell phone (or type the URL into your browser) for proof.

https://www.cardiovascularbusiness.com/topics/lipids-metabolic/americans-dying-because-cant-afford-insulin

PBMs have emerged from the sewers and are on a mission to maximize their shareholders' profits while systematically wiping out diabetics who cannot afford their insulin. The media offers abundant real-life examples documenting how diabetics are suffering at the hands of PBMs. The morbidity and mortality that are being inflicted upon individuals with diabetes who cannot afford their insulin co-pays is not acceptable. Additionally, there are countless millions of patients going without their HIV/AIDS medications, asthma inhalers, and other lifesaving drugs.

Here is a great informational video that explains why *your* medications are unaffordable:

https://www.youtube.com/watch?v=15IQO_jTMUM&feature=youtu.be

One of the key constructs of pharmacy is the Patient's Bill of Rights: all individuals are entitled to receive the right drug, prescribed to the right patient, in the right dose, via the right route of administration, prescribed for the right diagnosis. But the reader (you) will soon be receiving your medications via the mail, or maybe they will be dropped from the sky by drones. In either case, good luck getting the correct prescription or asking any questions of the actual pharmacist who filled your prescription. Good luck having any clue who was involved in filling your prescription or from what country the drugs and their ingredients may have originated. Currently the majority of active pharmaceutical ingredients (API) and finished pharmaceuticals are entering the global supply chain via China and India, where regulations are virtually nonexistent and quality assurance is routinely circumvented in order to maximize profits (DeNoon, 2008; "Safeguarding the U.S. Drug Supply," 2019). According to a special report by Reuters, brokers admit that an API made by an unregulated chemical company would cost less than one from a company that had a GMP [good manufacturing practices] certificate…"Different (API) grades have different prices. Sometimes we accept an order sheet and we happen to find a factory that can do it cheaper than our factory, we will outsource that to them and make a bigger margin"…In China there are few legal repercussions for broker firms who relabel or misrepresent products, and tracing counterfeit and substandard API is extremely difficult because there is no reliable API registry. "There are a lot of brokers who are relabeling API, which means you can't trace where the API comes from and that adds to the risk." (Lee, 2012)

Inferior foreign drugs have already killed many unsuspecting patients in the United States. It is highly probable that the generic drugs that are currently in your medicine cabinet were made in China or India and have *never* been inspected by the FDA. At this point, I wish to make a very clear distinction between my disapproval of the lack of governmental regulatory oversight of the pharmaceutical industry by foreign governments and my empathy and compassion for the great people of China, India, and other nations. As a matter of public health and national security, I feel compelled to make all persons aware that over 80 percent of the prescription drugs they are consuming are being manufactured overseas, in facilities that routinely ignore good manufacturing practices (GMP) and have no respect for the authority of the FDA.

When I worked as a chemist for RORER Pharmaceuticals in Fort Washington, Pennsylvania, in the 1980s, my job was to assure that GMP were being followed by conducting quality assurance and quality control tests on the formulation, stability, and potency of their flagship products Maalox and Ascriptin. Every batch of every finished drug was tested for its composition using high-performance liquid chromatography (HPLC). HPLC is accomplished with a laboratory machine that is used to identify and quantify the API in the sample being tested. It can also detect any contaminants that might be present. Each component is separated from the others and appears as a unique and measurable "peak" on a chromatogram.

I was also involved with long-term drug stability testing across a wide range of temperatures. Dissolution tests were also conducted, during which an Ascriptin tablet would be dropped into a water bath with a particular pH to simulate the acidity of a human stomach. Observations and measurements were recorded to make sure that the tablets could actually be expected to dissolve and be absorbed into systemic circulation. Each individual API and excipient (inactive ingredients such as binders, fillers, and coloring agents) that went into the recipe was cataloged and documented as to its sourcing and lot number.

In the 1980s I worked as a microbiology technician for McNeil Pharmaceutical in Spring House, Pennsylvania. I was in charge of conducting testing on the water supply for the entire manufacturing facility, while observing all GMP and SOP (standard operating procedures). My quality assurance work was instrumental in maintaining the microbiological integrity of the finished drug product that many thousands of consumers depended upon. Everything was always done exactly by the book—with the knowledge that FDA could walk in and conduct an unannounced (surprise!) inspection at any time in search of deviations from GMP.

Generic pharmaceutical firms in China and India have little fear of a surprise FDA inspection because they are thousands of miles away and are typically given up to twelve weeks' advance notice. Data integrity is frequently a concern when it comes to overseas pharmaceutical facilities. They can (and do) simply fudge all the manufacturing batch records and fabricate all the quality assurance and stability data. The notorious Indian pharma company Ranbaxy has proven how extremely simple it is to create an illusion of compliance, especially with so many years between FDA inspections, as well as advance warnings of such inspections. FDA has stated that "appropriate controls are not established over computerised systems…This is a repeat observation from the previous FDA inspection in 12/2012…Specifically the standalone computerised system controlling GC#6 does not have sufficient controls to prevent unauthorised access to, changes to, or omission of data files and folders (GAO-11-936T)." Essentially, when a quality assurance measure fails, workers can (and do) easily go back into the computer system and replace the data with whatever numbers they wish—magically creating passing laboratory results.

India, unlike China, means us no intentional harm economically or politically. Unequivocally, India's substandard medications are killing us, but despite its pharmaceutical quality control shortcomings, India is less of an existential threat to our national security than is China. India is our friend, and such an ally is never going to try to intentionally undermine us or send a nuclear missile in our direction. The government of India is focused on taking care of its own people and, unlike China, has no aspirations of global military and economic imperialism. A recent CNN documentary (May 2020) highlighted a huge military parade during which China showcased many thousands of troops, tanks, and an enormous array of road-mobile missiles capable of reaching every American military installation in the region, as well as long-range missiles that could accurately hit every American city. The Chinese Dongfeng-26 (DF-26) is an intermediate-range ballistic missile that has one purpose—to take out US aircraft carriers and other assets in the South China Sea or elsewhere in the region. The DF-26 is China's first conventional/nuclear missile that is capable of reaching Guam. Not only is China likely liable for unintentionally creating the deadly COVID-19 pandemic, but it has also evidently covered it up and possibly lied about the number of cases (Diamond, 2020). When hero Dr. Li Wenliang sounded the warning bell, he was silenced by the Chinese government. No one is saying that China intentionally unleashed the deadly contagion upon the world: "COVID-19 is a zoonosis just like many other contemporary viral diseases that presumably jumped from animals to humans. China has closed its wild animal markets in response to COVID-19" (Diamond, 2020). Nevertheless, according to a study published in March of 2020, the spread of COVID-19 cases could have been prevented if China had been transparent and acted responsibly (*WSJ*, 2020). Furthermore, China has a proven track record of stealing our intellectual property and has been accused of attempting to hack into US universities' and pharmaceutical and health care firms' databases to steal COVID-19 treatment and vaccine research data. If true, this would be a direct assault on American public health and our national security. According to the FBI, "This alleged activity is a significant threat to the U.S. response to the new coronavirus" (Sanger, 2020).

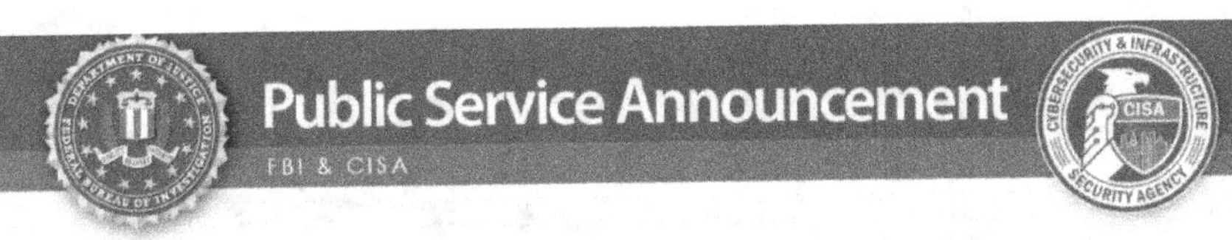

13 May 2020

People's Republic of China (PRC) Targeting of COVID-19 Research Organizations

The Federal Bureau of Investigation (FBI) and Cybersecurity and Infrastructure Security Agency (CISA) are issuing this announcement to raise awareness of the threat to COVID-19-related research. The FBI is investigating the targeting and compromise of U.S. organizations conducting COVID-19-related research by PRC-affiliated cyber actors and non-traditional collectors. These actors have been observed attempting to identify and illicitly obtain valuable intellectual property (IP) and public health data related to vaccines, treatments, and testing from networks and personnel affiliated with COVID-19-related research. The potential theft of this information jeopardizes the delivery of secure, effective, and efficient treatment options.

We should not be at the mercy of China or *any* outside player when it comes to the integrity of the medications that we depend on. Even if China and India both clean up their acts and begin to produce high-quality pharmaceuticals, our national security will still be at risk if outsiders continue to control the global drug supply chain. While the current supply chain interruption is totally due to COVID-19, it must serve as our public health 9/11. China can intentionally and arbitrarily stop shipping all API at any moment. The shelves of every pharmacy on the globe would rapidly become barren. The United States, including our military, would have no drugs, and our health care system would cease to function. So long as it controls the drug supply chain, China can easily take over the world without firing a shot.

Scan the QR code below to read the Bloomberg article on deadly generic Chinese drugs that are killing US citizens. This public health disaster has been exacerbated by the supply chain disruptions being caused by the COVID-19 pandemic. Thanks to the coronavirus, we are now experiencing critical shortages of the very same inferior nonbioequivalent generic pharmaceutical products that have been killing us anyway. We can't live with these toxic Chinese-manufactured drugs, and we can't live without these toxic Chinese-manufactured drugs! FDA is our gatekeeper, our protector, and our savior. Read the article below to understand why we must give FDA more resources so that it can protect our pharmaceutical supply chain from deadly foreign contamination as effectively as possible.

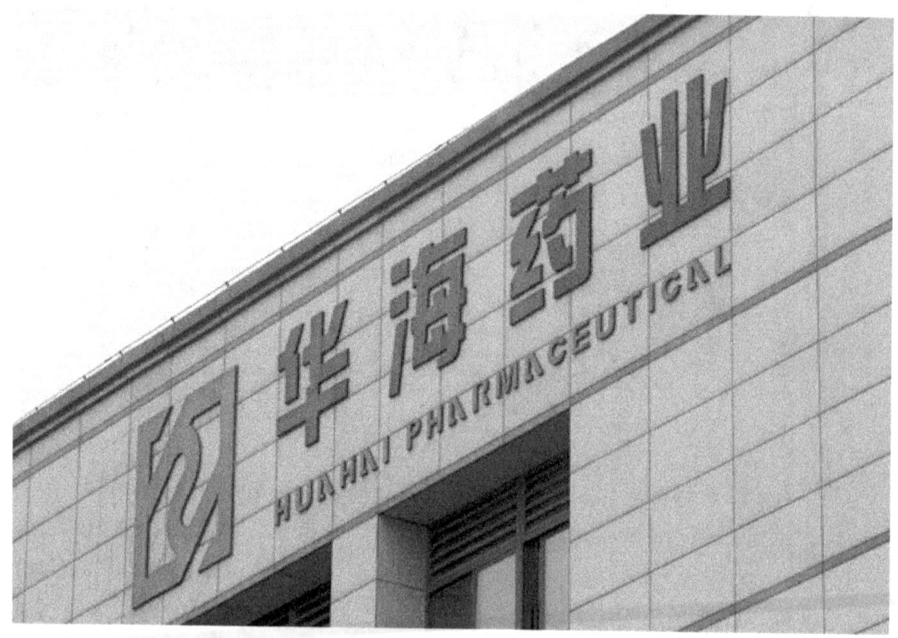

https://www.bloomberg.com/news/features/2019-09-12/
how-carcinogen-tainted-generic-drug-valsartan-got-past-the-fda

Mr. Jun Du

Executive Vice President

Zhejiang Huahai Pharmaceutical Co., Ltd.

Coastal Industrial Zone, Chuannan No. 1 Branch No. 9

Donghai Fifth Avenue, Linhai, Taizhou Zhejiang 317016

CHINA

Dear Mr. Du:

The U.S. Food and Drug Administration (FDA) inspected your drug manufacturing facility, Zhejiang Huahai Pharmaceutical Co., Ltd., located at Coastal Industrial Zone, Chuannan No. 1 Branch No. 9, Donghai Fifth Avenue, Linhai, Taizhou Zhejiang, from July 23 to August 3, 2018.

This warning letter summarizes significant deviations from current good manufacturing practice (CGMP) for active pharmaceutical ingredients (API).

Remember the days when patients like you, the reader, had access to a corner drugstore pharmacist on whom you could rely for free advice and for the correct medication, manufactured right here in the United States, under the full force and protection of the FDA?

Community pharmacy is facing an uphill battle for survival against the combined forces of pharmacy benefit managers, mail-order mammoths, and behemoth chain drugstores. As more community pharmacies are forced to close, Americans are rapidly losing their quick access to lifesaving drugs that they need for survival. Instead, there are long waits at chain drugstores (and increased risk of exposures to germs, including COVID-19) or eternal waits for arrival of mail-order drug deliveries.

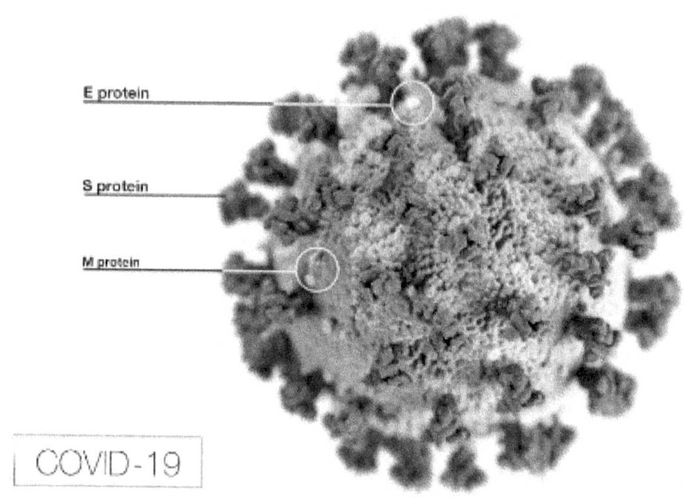

As the novel coronavirus rages on, it is not the large chain drugstores or the mail-order drug houses that are stepping up to save the day. Instead, small community pharmacies are coming to the rescue, just as they have for the last one-hundred-plus years, with free same-day home delivery of lifesaving medications to senior citizens and other high-risk patients who cannot afford to venture out into the unsafe environment.

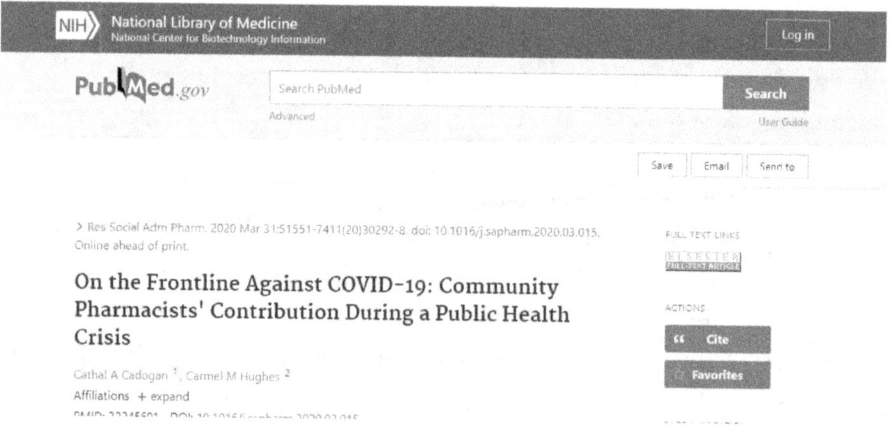

Meanwhile, FDA is at the mercy of rogue foreign individuals, unlicensed suppliers, manufacturers, and governments who continue to put profits ahead of safety, breaching our supply chain with second-rate ingredients that are killing us. Remember the days before FDA was there to protect us, and people routinely died from unregulated toxic drugs? Remember the days when drugs were manufactured in the United States by licensed manufacturers using pure, FDA-approved ingredients that actually cured sick people rather than contributed to patient deaths? Do not underestimate the magnitude of this public health disaster. People are dying daily, domestically and globally, from filthy and putrefied pharmaceuticals. For example, Kelesidis and Falagas (2015) report that in Africa and Asia, the prevalence of low-quality antimicrobial pharmaceuticals is as high as 50 percent in some studies. Similarly, the number of counterfeit drugs appearing in Europe and the United States has increased exponentially. India, China, and Thailand are the sources for the majority of counterfeit drugs that flood Asia, Africa, Europe, and North America (Kelesidis & Falagas, 2015). These fake drugs find their way into the US supply chain through repackagers, importers, and internet pharmacies, directly affecting our national security.

Take a good look at today's global drug environment and watch sadly as the two protectors of the pharmaceutical world—the community pharmacist and FDA—are helpless as we devolve back to the days of an unregulated Wild West drug free-for-all.

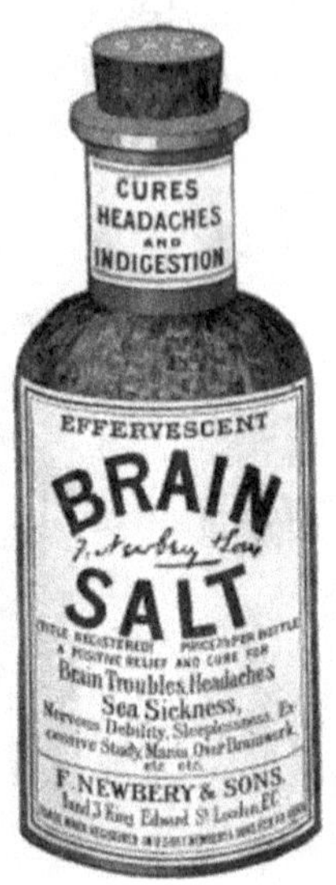

We are gradually returning to the patent medicine era, a drug circus with tainted and misbranded drugs flowing freely and harming people indiscriminately. The community pharmacist and FDA are the only safety nets between the American people and the exponential number of deadly drugs that are pouring across our borders and into our medicine cabinets. Blockchain technology allows for the recording of transactions across a network of users. When fully implemented by Big Pharma, blockchain may alleviate—but not cure—the problem (Roberts, 2017). A simple internet search yields numerous websites offering countless Chinese API vendors that are not GMP certified. Any amateur counterfeiter can easily visit online trade boards like Alibaba and purchase whatever API he or she needs directly from China, mix it up in a bathtub with an oar, and ship it globally.

https://www.alibaba.com/showroom/alibaba-pharmaceuticals.html

FOREWORD

Health Care Roulette has been many years in the making. In its original iteration, as *Rx Roulette*, the focus was primarily on how adulterated and misbranded foreign drugs present deadly dangers to the integrity of the legitimate pharmaceutical supply chain. This phenomenon still holds very true, as impure and falsely labeled pharmaceuticals continue to flow into the United States from China, India, Mexico, and Canada. There are well-documented cases that will be discussed in *Health Care Roulette* of US citizens dying from filthy imported drug products (DeNoon, 2008). To make matters even more complex, the COVID-19 outbreak has brought global pharmaceutical manufacturing to a standstill, creating catastrophic shortages of almost every medication, including antimalarials, bronchodilators, antibiotics, and antivirals.

The influx of contaminated counterfeit drugs is directly connected to another phenomenon that is making health care headlines and demands the immediate attention of the general public. A new animal called the pharmacy benefit manager (PBM) has reared its ugly head, committing unconscionable malfeasance that strikes at the very heart of our health care system. PBMs are the nexus for the astronomical drug pricing that is plaguing society. The ambiguous role that PBMs play in our complex multipayer, multiplayer health care system confuses even seasoned advocates of public health and well-being. Scan the QR code below to make sure you are not overpaying for you medications:

https://www.youtube.com/watch?v=h2_yDTU5kJw&feature=youtu.be

Americans pay more for their prescription drugs than any other nation in the world (Bradley & Taylor, 2013). It's a hard pill to swallow when you can't afford to fill your prescriptions. It is an atrocity that working-class people have to choose between taking their lifesaving prescription drugs and paying the rent (Cefalu et al., 2018). In his Rose Garden speech of May 2018, the president of the United States specifically took aim at PBMs as being part of the broken system: "We're very much eliminating the middlemen. The middlemen became very, very rich. Right? Whoever those middlemen were—and a lot of people never even figured it out—they're rich. They won't be so rich anymore." The president went on to say, "Our plan will end the dishonest double-dealing that allows the middlemen to pocket rebates and discounts that should be passed on to consumers and patients" (Trump, 2018). Disappointingly, there was no follow-up action from Washington as of the spring of 2020.

A formulary is a list of medications that are covered by the insurance company. Formularies typically contain various tiers that are associated with different levels of preferred products. The formulary and corresponding co-pay for each drug in each tier on the formulary are typically dictated by PBMs. The highest tier in the formulary has the lowest co-pay for the patient, and the lowest tier has the highest co-pay. Formularies typically have three tiers, with first-tier drugs being categorized as "preferred" and thus having lower co-pays. Second- and third-tier drugs have higher co-pays and typically require prior authorizations. PBMs are for-profit intermediaries that operate clandestinely between Big Pharma, insurance companies, pharmacies, and patients. PBMs operate in a nontransparent manner and collect fees from all parties involved, including the pharmaceutical manufacturers (rebates), pharmacies (claim transmission fees, direct and indirect remuneration fees), insurers, and patients (co-pays). Formulary decisions revolve around PBM rebates and kickbacks, not necessarily what is medically advisable for the patient's well-being. Big Pharma is blackmailed into paying off the PBMs for pole position on the formulary, thus forcing manufacturers to keep raising their list prices. The net price is what the manufacturer retains after getting fleeced by the PBM. All the while, Scrooge-like PBMs calculate patient co-pays based on the list price rather than on the discounted price after rebates. Since higher co-pays translate into higher out-of-pocket expenses, many patients must refrain from filling their prescriptions (Austvoll-Dahlgren et al., 2008; Kang et al., 2018). Due to their high costs, PBMs typically place specialty pharmaceuticals among the highest-tiered co-payments, creating disparities in access to the most vulnerable populations, which are disproportionately affected by the social determinants of health. Hence, persons with less desirable employment and working conditions, lower education and literacy levels, and lower socioeconomic status are more likely to be unable to take their medication as prescribed due to cost. These individuals will not fill their prescriptions and will be more likely to suffer disability and death (Austvoll-Dahlgen et al., 2008; Gourzoulidis et al., 2017; Tamblyn et al., 2001). Insulin co-pays in excess of $1,000 are not uncommon. For patients with type 1 diabetes, this means that they will quickly develop diabetic ketoacidosis and die if they cannot afford to purchase their insulin. Disgracefully, almost one hundred years after the discovery of insulin, diabetics are dying every day in the United States at the hands of greedy PBMs.

The Flow of Payment for Brand-Name Drugs Is Complex

Excludes federally mandated rebate programs

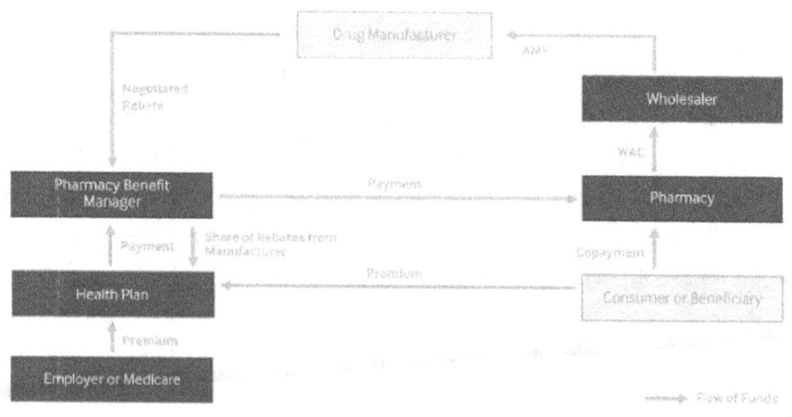

Note: AMP = Average Manufacturer Price, WAC = Wholesale Acquisition Cost.
Source: Congressional Budget Office.

PBMs typically blame Big Pharma for high out-of-pocket drug expenses, and vice versa. Big Pharma is currently racing to find treatments, cures, and vaccines for the deadly COVID-19. PBMs are nothing more than middlemen that siphon money out of the health care system and out of your wallet in the form of unaffordable pharmacy co-pays.

https://www.pbs.org/newshour/show/
do-prescription-drug-middlemen-help-keep-prices-high

This money is being stolen from the hardworking stakeholders (patients, payers, and providers) and is being redirected to line the pockets of the investing shareholders. In actuality, these funds should be redistributed to the enrollees in the form of lower out-of-pocket costs. PBMs should be held accountable to the highest level of social responsibility, but instead they are shareholder driven and represent a major conflict of interest across the continuum. PBMs should be nonprofit entities and obligated to show complete transparency of all financials. Insurers and PBMs have a moral and social obligation to make prescription drugs affordable to all by putting their patients' best interests ahead of those of their shareholders—and they should have a legal obligation to do so as well. Instead, it's all about Wall Street and maximizing the price of the stock by intentionally inflating prescription drug prices and pharmacy co-pays. PBMs weaponize drug cost sharing in an attempt to reduce third-party-payer drug expenditures and to combat moral hazard by deterring "unnecessary or marginal utilization" (Austvoll-Dahlgren et al., 2008). These unaffordable co-pays, especially in the case of vulnerable populations (the elderly and the poor), cause patients to be unable to afford to take their medications as prescribed due to cost, resulting in medication nonadherence. Medication nonadherence, in turn, results in negative health outcomes, including significant morbidity and mortality (Austvoll-Dahlgen et al., 2008; Gourzoulidis et al., 2017; Tamblyn et al., 2001).

The COVID-19 pandemic, for example, is disproportionately affecting the elderly and the poor, both of which are also high-risk groups for diabetes. The elderly are typically on Medicare, while the poor are usually covered by Medicaid (welfare). Additionally, there is a huge pool of 1099 self-employed independent contract workers who have no health insurance whatsoever. Poor minorities and the elderly, particularly those with comorbid conditions such as diabetes and asthma, are being wiped out by COVID-19 at higher rates than the general population (ADA, 2020; Galvin; 2020; *Morbidity and Mortality Weekly*, April 2020). If we connect the dots, we can observe a correlation between intentional *PBM-induced* prescription drug cost unaffordability, medication nonadherence among elderly and poor minority populations, and resulting negative health outcomes. There has been well-documented media coverage of the disproportionately of COVID-19 deaths among African Americans, Latinos, and the elderly.

Caveat Emptor: Canadian Knockoff Drugs Will Knock You Off

Insurance premiums can be thought of as what it costs you to *have* insurance. Deductibles are what it costs you "out of pocket" before your insurance actually kicks in. Finally, co-pays are what it costs you to finally be able to *use* your insurance when you really need it. Unaffordable premiums, deductibles, and co-pays inflicted by avaricious insurance companies and PBMs are forcing our desperate senior citizens and working-class persons to unwittingly purchase counterfeit nonbioequivalent drugs from rogue online internet sources, often disguised as legitimate "Canadian" pharmacy storefronts in US strip malls. Most commonly, these pharmacies (which are actually not licensed pharmacies but rather middlemen facilitator storefronts that are not even staffed by pharmacists) accept prescriptions from patients. The medications, which are not stocked on the premises, are then supposedly shipped from Canada to the patient's front door. There are also many internet-based "Canadian" pharmacies that cater to the American public. Even if the medications actually ship from Canada, they are most likely manufactured elsewhere with unknown ingredients in sloppy, underregulated environments. The following video link is a must watch to protect you and your loved ones from counterfeit Canadian knockoffs before they kill you (Levitt, 2017).

https://www.abcactionnews.com/money/consumer/taking-action-for-you/
popular-online-canadian-pharmacy-ordered-to-shutdown-over-counterfeit-medicine

Many policy influencers and politicians are touting the benefits of cheaper overseas imports. The Safe Importation Action Plan calls for allowing the importation of drugs originally intended for foreign markets. "Canadian" drugs would flow freely across the border, as would inferior foreign versions of FDA-approved products. The plan suggests there would be no additional risks to public safety because manufacturing records would be periodically audited.

https://www.cbsnews.com/news/ranbaxy-whistleblower-reveals-how-he-exposed-massive-
pharmaceutical-fraud/

Yet the 2019 *Report on Drug Safety* issued by the Government Accountability Office (GAO) notes that foreign pharmaceutical manufacturers have ample time to falsify manufacturing records because FDA gives them at least twelve weeks' advance notice of inspections prior to arrival. The Ranbaxy misadventure, as mentioned in my previous edition of *Health Care Roulette*, clearly illustrates that Americans' health and well-being are at risk from inferior foreign nonbioequivalent drugs. Eban (2019) has identified and described yet another example of data falsification, this time by Indian drug manufacturer Indoco Remedies. The actual FDA warning letter to Indoco can be viewed by following the link below:

https://www.fda.gov/inspections-compliance-enforcement-and-criminal-investigations/
warning-letters/indoco-remedies-limited-575313-07162019

The infamous Ranbaxy calamity made headlines in the *Wall Street Journal* and dates back to 2013, while the Indoco case occurred much more recently, in 2019, clearly illustrating that foreign pharmaceutical manufacturing fraud is still a significant problem. A Google search for FDA warning letters yields an infinite number of additional examples of drug problems originating in China and India. The take-home message here is that there is no such thing as a Safe Importation

Action Plan because foreign drugs circumvent FDA scrutiny, are not bioequivalent to the innovator products, and will never be safe for human consumption.

https://www.fda.gov/news-events/speeches-fda-officials/
hhs-media-briefing-safe-importation-action-plan-07312019

Few realize the deadly consequences associated with knockoff drugs. To many, drug counterfeiting is considered to be an act of terrorism against public health as well as an act of economic sabotage (Lewis, 2009). FDA lacks complete and accurate information on foreign drug manufacturers, distributors, and other participants in the complex global flow of pharmaceuticals, thus making it impossible to guarantee the safety of the drug supply chain. The *Wall Street Journal* referenced a study conducted by the Alliance for Safe Online Pharmacies in which 55 percent of consumers said they have or would purchase medications online (Reddy, 2018). The very same article shows a picture of a mother holding a snapshot of her son, who died after ingesting a counterfeit drug obtained on the internet. Photos of the drug show that while it appeared almost identical to the real brand-name product, it actually contained a lethal dose of fentanyl (Reddy, 2018).

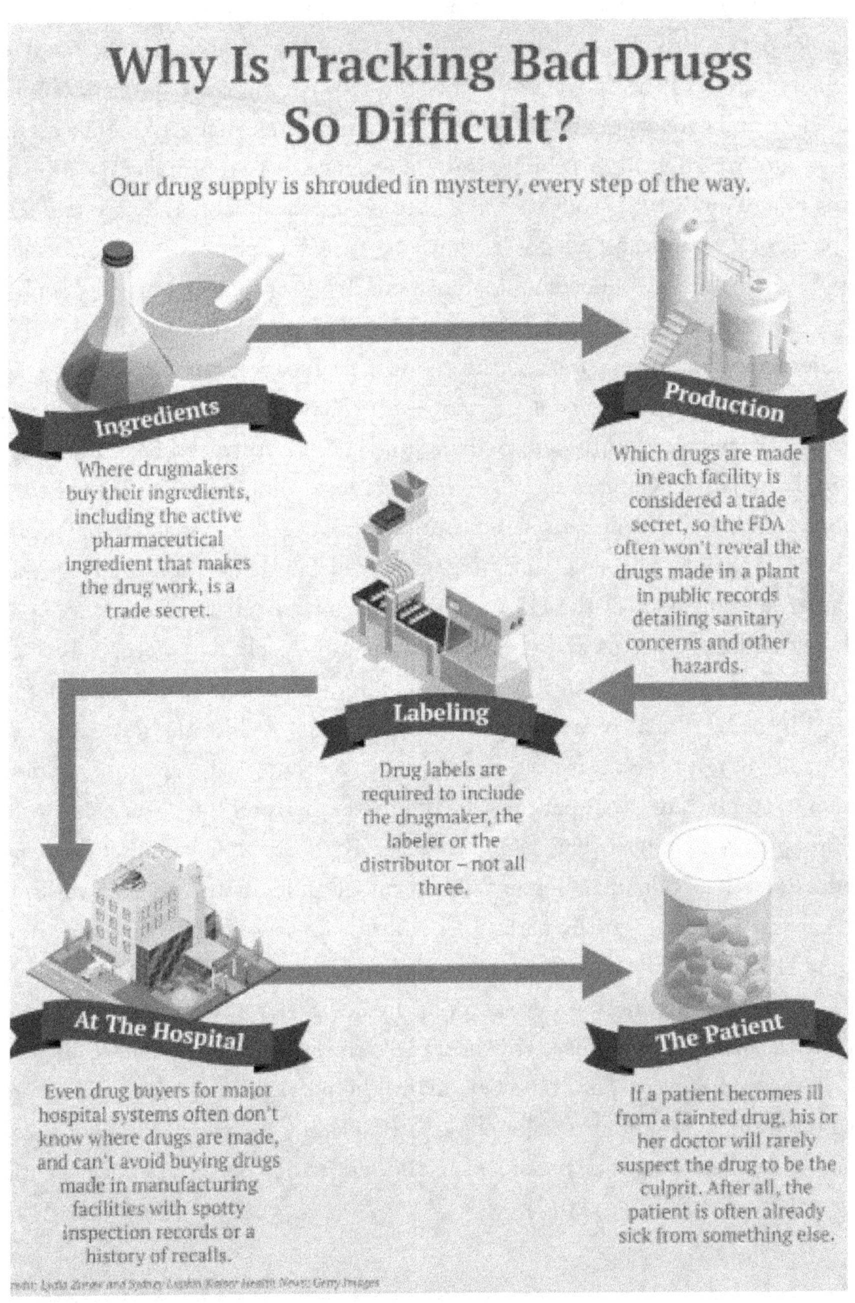
Why Is Tracking Bad Drugs So Difficult?
Our drug supply is shrouded in mystery, every step of the way.
Ingredients
Where drugmakers buy their ingredients, including the active pharmaceutical ingredient that makes the drug work, is a trade secret.
Production
Which drugs are made in each facility is considered a trade secret, so the FDA often won't reveal the drugs made in a plant in public records detailing sanitary concerns and other hazards.
Labeling
Drug labels are required to include the drugmaker, the labeler or the distributor – not all three.
At The Hospital
Even drug buyers for major hospital systems often don't know where drugs are made, and can't avoid buying drugs made in manufacturing facilities with spotty inspection records or a history of recalls.
The Patient
If a patient becomes ill from a tainted drug, his or her doctor will rarely suspect the drug to be the culprit. After all, the patient is often already sick from something else.
Credit: Lydia Zuraw and Sydney Lupkin/Kaiser Health News; Getty Images

The drug supply chain is vulnerable to accidental or intentional sabotage and includes not only the finished drug products that end up in our bathroom medicine cabinets but all of the active and supposedly inactive ingredients that comprise completed pharmaceuticals. *Bioequivalence* is a term in pharmacokinetics used to assess the expected in vivo biological equivalence of two proprietary preparations of a drug. If two products are said to be bioequivalent, they are expected to be, for all intents and purposes, the same. Any breach of the pharmaceutical supply chain can introduce nonbioequivalent drugs onto our pharmacy shelves. There are abundant contemporary examples: The blood pressure drugs valsartan, losartan, and irbesartan and the stomach medication ranitidine, along with countless others, were recently discovered to have been adulterated with the deadly carcinogen N-Nitrosodimethylamine (NDMA), traced back to unregulated, lackadaisical Chinese suppliers that have zero comprehension of the Federal Food, Drug, and Cosmetic Act and routinely cut corners to make fatter profits. While China does have its China Food and Drug Administration (CFDA), there is no true equivalent of the US FDA in China or anywhere else in the world. Underregulated pharma and chemical companies freely do whatever they can to maximize revenue, even if it means feeding uninspected, nonbioequivalent drugs into the global pharmaceutical supply chain. While the government of China might not be *endorsing* the counterfeit drug trade, it is certainly not doing much to ameliorate the situation. China puts the onus on the buyer to only deal with registered Chinese drug producers (Lewis, 2009). It is vital that the reader understand that "Canadian" drugs are often made anonymously in China or India, perhaps in someone's filthy bathtub, with inferior ingredients that have never been FDA inspected. According to a Reuters report, "A key regulatory weakness in China is the distinction between pharmaceutical and chemical companies. While the former are regulated by the CFDA, the latter, making everything from sweeteners to solvents, are not. Yet, many chemical companies also churn out drug ingredients, exploiting a loophole by describing the products as chemicals, which they are, rather than the more specific designation of Active Pharmaceutical Ingredients (API)" (Lee, 2012).

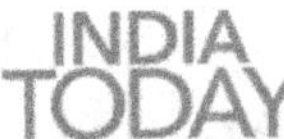

NEWS •LIVE TV **INDIA TODAY** APP MA

HOME | VIDEOS | CORONAVIRUS OUTBREAK | INDIA | MOVIES | TRENDING | TECH | SPORTS | BINGE WATCH | LIFES

News / India /

As workers skip duty, truckers refuse to move amid lockdown, pharma units warn of medicine shortage

The lockdown and curfew in many states has broken the medicine supply chain. The pharma unit owners say they were compelled to stop manufacturing activity as some ancillary units that make foil, packaging material and printers have shut down.

Under the stressors of the COVID-19 pandemic, China's pharmaceutical manufacturing came to a grinding halt. India, which depends on China for most of its pharmaceutical ingredients, also stopped making and exporting drugs. For example, there was a brief period of time in which the antimalarial drug hydroxy-chloroquine was being publicly touted as a potential remedy for COVID-19, until clinical studies suggested it was a potentially very dangerous drug. Meanwhile, India immediately halted all exports of hydroxychloroquine (and many other criti-cal drugs including metronidazole, chloramphenicol, erythromycin, neomycin, clindamycin, acetaminophen, acyclovir, and some vitamins) so that they could stockpile medications for their own citizens. It was not unreasonable for India to put its own citizens ahead of the rest of the world considering the severity and uncertainty of the global environmental situation due to COVID-19, but it leaves the United States in a precarious situation. Although research is still ongoing, the possible adverse side effect profile of hydroxychloroquine has so far prevented its widespread use to treat COVID-19. But if science determines that the benefits are deemed to outweigh the possible risks, the drug may fall back into favor.

Making matters even worse, antimalarial drugs such as hydroxychloroquine are among the most frequently counterfeited drugs in the developing world (Kelesidis & Falagas, 2015). How ironic would it be if @POTUS, who has publicly acknowledged taking hydroxychloroquine prophylactically, was unwittingly taking a nonbioequivalent Chinese or Indian counterfeit knockoff drug! "In India, the penalties for making and selling counterfeit medications are minimal, the convictions are rare, and the profits are enormous" (the Center for Safe Internet Pharmacies, 2019). The previous example clearly illustrates our dependence on inferior foreign-made nonbioequivalent drugs. As factories in China and India shut down from the coronavirus, US pharmacies quickly lost access to innumerable pharmaceuticals, including many critical blood pressure pills, Alzheimer's disease tablets (donepezil, for example), cholesterol medications (statins), and antibiotics. Virtually all cephalosporin antibiotics, vitamin C, ibuprofen, acetaminophen, and hydrocortisone originate in China. The bottle of penicillin that I recently examined on a local pharmacy shelf was made in India, as were all the losartan, valacyclovir, ursodiol, fenofibrate, montelukast, pantoprazole, fluoxetine, amlodipine, and warfarin. Warfarin is an extremely dangerous narrow therapeutic index (NTI) anticoagulant drug that can easily cause massive uncontrolled bleeding, especially if it is nonbioequivalent to the innovator product. Most patients at the pharmacy counter have no idea that their drugs are originating from all over the world. In many cases, the pharmacist does not know, either, because the stock bottles of medication make mention of the distributor but do not always disclose the identity or location of the drug manufacturer. Despite the fact that these drugs are produced in faraway lands, with no appreciation of good manufacturing practices (GMP), we literally cannot live without them. The worldwide shortage of drugs precipitated by the coronavirus should be sounding our wake-up call: America needs to reclaim its generic pharmaceutical industry and stop being held hostage by the undiversified and insecure global supply chain. We must never be caught off guard again!

I strongly agree with the coronavirus plan put forth by Senator Marco Rubio because it also should improve the quality of the pharmaceuticals we are ingesting. First off, Rubio points out that the Department of Defense and the FDA do not know the volume of API sourced from China. Rubio's bill would mandate that the drug manufacturers' annual reports disclose the volume of API sourced from each supplier in the prior year. This resource will allow the FDA to keep tabs on our degree of dependence on China and to identify potential drug shortages before they manifest. I also concur with Rubio's proposal to allow the VA to determine a drug's country of origin based on where the API was sourced. Rubio's statement that "the U.S. runs the risk of losing important components of its medical supply chain to China's government-backed industry" rings true to me (rubio.senate.gov). Furthermore, from a pharmacist's perspective, I am petrified to dispense drugs from China and India to my patients and family.

Our vulnerability to and dependence on foreign suppliers is putting our national security at risk, and it extends far beyond the pharmaceutical industry. Everything from medicinal products to ventilators, face masks, and other personal protective equipment (PPE) has been unavailable to first responders and medical personnel. How is it that we must turn to China to purchase the PPE to save us from the virus that China released, albeit accidently? At the time of publication of this book, heroes (doctors, nurses, and first responders) are all falling victim to COVID-19. Ventilators are being rationed, offered only to those patients who have the best chance for survival, leaving countless, nameless others, including those affected by health disparities, to die alone. Shortages also abound among drugs required to treat patients on ventilators—namely, sedatives, analgesics, anesthetics, and muscle relaxants.

The social determinants of health are, disgracefully, shining through once again, as African Americans and Latinos are falling victim to COVID-19 in disproportionally high numbers. Furthermore, these very same populations are also at higher risk for diabetes, which in turn has been associated with worse COVID-19 outcomes (ADA, 2019). Often, persons with diabetes suffer social and health disparities that render them unable to afford to take their medications due to cost. These individuals, consequently, do not manage their diabetes well and often experience fluctuating blood sugars. As such, they are generally at risk for a number of diabetes-related complications. Having heart disease or other complications in addition to diabetes could worsen the chance of getting seriously ill from COVID-19, like other viral infections, because the body's ability to fight off an infection is compromised. Importantly, COVID-19 is a much deadlier pathogen than the seasonal flu, especially for people with diabetes. People who already have diabetes-related health problems are likely to have worse outcomes if they contract COVID-19 than people with diabetes who are otherwise healthy. Consequently, all of the standard precautions to avoid infection that have been widely recommended by the CDC are even more important when dealing with the potentially deadly COVID-19 (Diclemente et al., 2013; Gourzoulidis et al., 2017; Tamblyn et al., 2001).

The world has not seen a pandemic of this magnitude since the Spanish flu of 1918, which killed upward of one hundred million people globally. From now on, we need to look at the world from a public health perspective. It's all about prevention and preparedness at every level, from disease prevention to creating surge capacity by stockpiling medications, medical supplies, and generators in case pandemics or other disasters occur. Individual households need to have at least three months' worth of medication, food, and water on hand at all times, rotating the stock to avoid spoilage. It makes no difference whether it's a hurricane, the plague, or another terrorist attack. We don't want to be fighting over the last loaf of bread at the corner store.

Every hospital must have a full-time disaster response team as well as stockpiles of ventilators and other mechanical devices, PPE (gloves, gowns, facemasks, etc.), disinfectants, medications, and needles and syringes for medication and vaccine administration. Vaccines, antibiotics, antivirals, cardiac drugs, anticoagulants, and other essentials, including food, need to be stored in bulk, consumed as indicated, and rotated accordingly. It is not unreasonable to construct separate "backup" hospital wings and secure storage areas stocked with a strategic reserve of equipment and medications. Mock disaster drills should be done quarterly, as well as inspections, cleaning, and preventive maintenance of all equipment. Upon each hospital's reaccreditation by the Joint Commission (JCAHO), surge capacity and stockpile review and inspection by JCAHO surveyors should be included. At the organizational level, corporations (large and small) should be mandated by the government to have emergency plans in place and enough PPE for their staff in case of an acute disaster or a chronic eruption such as a second wave of COVID-19. Scientists have already noted increasing cases, as quarantine and lockdown measures have been relaxed in many locations (Holcombe, 2020).

Essential businesses may want to stockpile (and rotate) bottled water, food, and other consumable supplies for their staff. The last place I want to be is fighting in the supermarket aisle over the last roll of toilet paper, as has been commonplace with the shortages created by the coronavirus pandemic. Municipal, state, and federal governments should be investing billions of dollars into warehousing all of the above emergency supplies, especially critical pharmaceuticals. There should be multiple secured warehouses in multiple secured locations in every state—complete with staffers (civilian and military), inspectors, and federal armed guards who will not hesitate to protect the staffers and the stockpiles. Nothing should ever be wasted: unused foods and other consumer items can regularly be sold off to the public at a discount or donated to food banks a few months before their expiration dates while being continuously replenished to maintain the national stockpile. Furthermore, US firms should be given financial incentives to manufacture these critical supplies right here at home so that no foreign nations can pull our strings.

The Defense Production Act was activated by the president in May of 2020 to help replenish the national stockpile, which was "severely depleted" during the H1N1 outbreak in 2009 and was never replenished (King, 2020). We don't have to wait for a once-in-a-hundred-years plague to use these stockpiles. There are hurricanes, earthquakes, wildfires, and other natural and manmade catastrophes occurring regularly. COVID-19, despite the gradual reopening of the country and the world, is not going away anytime soon. We will need to draw upon these resources frequently and continuously—and the federal government is willing to cover the initial supply and replenishment costs through "loans and other financing that are limited to create, maintain, protect, expand, or restore domestic industrial base capabilities" (King, 2020). This is a small price to pay for avoiding another catastrophic failure and a repeat performance of the current environmental disaster we are facing. Furthermore, these stockpiled supplies need to be purchased, when possible, only from US companies that employ US workers and manufacture on US soil. When it comes to purchasing medications and critical supplies, buying from China is tantamount to spinning the roulette wheel. As a pharmacist, I believe that every pharmacy should stockpile at least three months' worth of critical medications, PPE, and other necessary supplies— at least until US manufacturers can reclaim the health care industry as their own once again. Every patient should always have a sufficient personal backup supply of all critical medications for himself or herself and all family members, including pets. Hopefully, the new lower corporate tax rate (down to 21 percent from 35 percent) announced by the president on May 7, 2020, will result in the United States' generic drug manufacturing industry roaring back to life. When it comes to essential supplies, we have to make American and buy American in order to protect our health, our economy, and national security.

https://khn.org/news/how-tainted-drugs-reach-market-make-patients-sicker/

In addition to the API that comprise each drug, there are binders, fillers, colors, and other excipients contained in the finished product. The FDA website details many examples of filthy, nonbioequivalent drugs that have been identified in the drug supply chain. FDA is our guardian, and I do not fault it. Still, the GAO reported that FDA does not have a true count on how many foreign drug establishments are manufacturing drugs for the US market. What is even scarier is that each of these foreign establishments often outsources individual steps in the global manufacturing process to other unknown, unlicensed subcontractors and suppliers of raw materials located on the other side of the world. Many have never registered with FDA and do not even have a clue what the acronym *GMP* stands for. FDA does not have the capacity to monitor every shipment of API and excipients that come out of China, India, or anywhere else. Additionally, the majority of pharmaceuticals that are manufactured in India are made from Chinese ingredients (Grant & Taplin, 2020). Consequently, all US citizens are playing a potentially deadly game of prescription roulette every time they ingest doses of imported nonbioequivalent generic medications. You don't have to take my word for it—do a Google search for the government publication GAO-11-936T and see for yourself, or just follow the QR and/or URL below.

https://www.gao.gov/products/GAO-11-936T

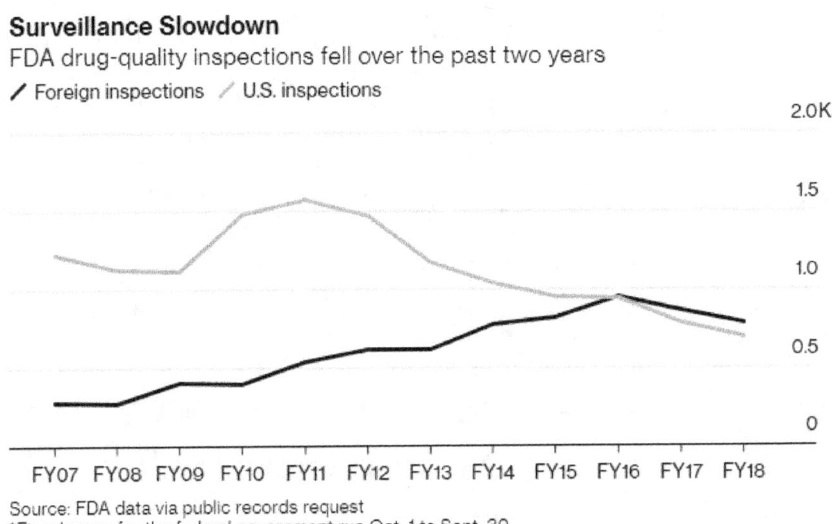

Fake drugs could be subpotent, containing little or none of the intended active ingredient. A prime example of this was the counterfeit chemotherapy drug Avastin, which entered the US drug supply chain through "Canadian" pharmacies. FDA lab tests concluded that "at least one batch of a counterfeit version of Avastin contained no active ingredient" (Rockoff, 2012). Cancer patients who received fake Avastin stood no chance and potentially lost their lives earlier than would have otherwise been the case due to receiving this inactive product. If not for the discovery of the counterfeit drug, the disease would have been assumed to be the cause of death. If you visit the website www.CanadaDrugs.com, you will see the outcome of the federal investigation regarding this deadly counterfeiting scheme (Weaver & Whalen, 2012).

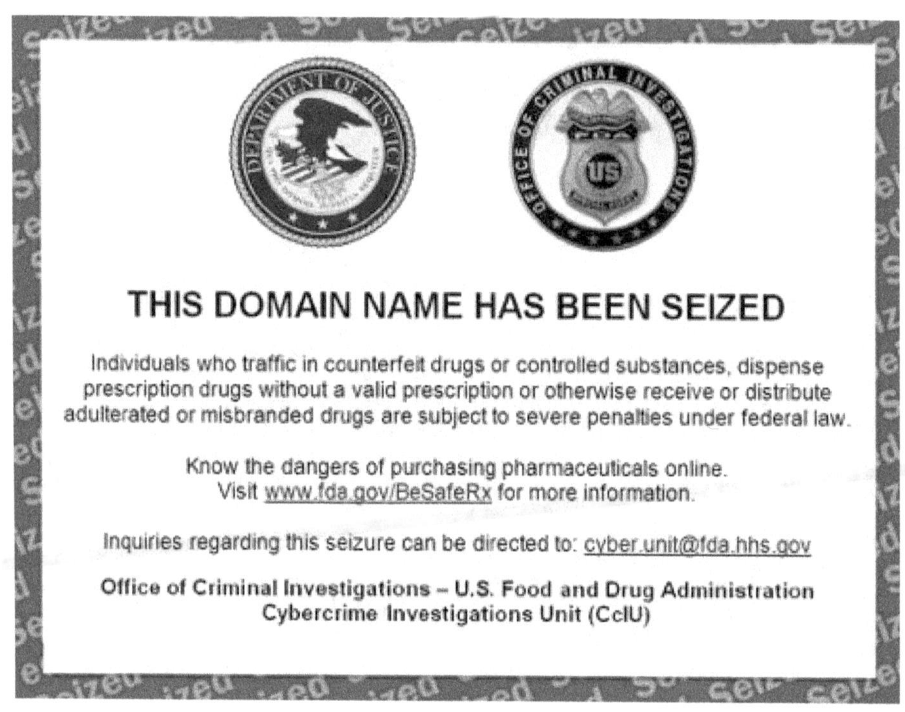

www.CanadaDrugs.com

https://www.safemedicines.org/wp-content/uploads/2015/08/CanadaDrugs-Indictment1.pdf

On the other hand, the product may be superpotent, containing potentially toxic or deadly quantities of the active ingredient. Hundreds of thousands of counterfeit pills, some containing deadly amounts of fentanyl, have been introduced into the US drug markets, exacerbating the US opioid crisis. The Drug Enforcement Administration released a report identifying a higher fentanyl presence and associated overdose deaths than at any time since the drug's creation in 1959. Fentanyl is used legitimately to treat severe pain and is usually dispensed in the form of transdermal patches, which release a specific dose of the drug into the body via skin absorption.

While this book is obviously very critical of the underregulated Chinese and Indian pharmaceutical industries, it is not targeting the individual citizens of China or India. It is the lack of government regulation and enforcement, not the hardworking people of China and India, that is to blame for the adulterated and misbranded drugs that are laden with contaminants and grossness. Chinese citizens are just as afraid of taking fake drugs as anyone else is. They suffer just like the rest of the world from taking counterfeits that don't work or are dangerous (Lewis, 2009). Meanwhile, naive US citizens are caught up in a high-stakes game of health care roulette, and it behooves the reader to visit the FDA's website and heed the warnings against purchasing drugs that circumvent the safety net of FDA and come from anonymous, unregulated sources on the other side of the world. An important link to FDA warning is provided here:

https://www.fda.gov/drugs/resourcesforyou/ucm078918.htm

Clandestine laboratories in China are mass-producing fentanyl and fentanyl-related compounds and selling them to drug-trafficking groups in Mexico, Canada, and the United States. Clandestine pill-press operations also occur in the United States. Counterfeit fentanyl pills often resemble the authentic medications they are intended to mimic, and the presence of fentanyl is only detected upon laboratory analysis. Oxycodone alone is culpable for countless opioid overdose deaths by respiratory depression. If someone expecting to take an oxycodone pill unexpectedly ingests a superpotent counterfeit containing fentanyl, the risk for respiratory depression and death increases greatly. In fact, oral fentanyl usually kills instantaneously. Similarly, if a heroin addict inadvertently injects a fentanyl-laced counterfeit, death will be swift. In addition to being deadly to users, fentanyl poses a lethal threat to first responders and law enforcement, as a lethal dose of fentanyl or the superpotent carfentanil can be accidentally inhaled or absorbed through the skin.

The health care environment is a continuum of dynamic events that changes frequently. Contemporary issues such as the COVID-19 pandemic, the diabetes pandemic, the opioid and vaping epidemics, and illegal foreign drug importation are simultaneously killing us off prematurely. It would take a team of mathematicians to calculate the total number of otherwise preventable daily deaths that are occurring. Senior citizens and all citizens should no longer be forced to make the life-or-death choice between purchasing imported inferior medications and putting food on their tables. Scan the QR code below to learn how to stop making the PBMs rich.

https://www.youtube.com/watch?v=h2_yDTU5kJw&feature=youtu.be

Big Pharma brings investment in research and development to the table and increases Americans' quality of life and longevity. If Big Pharma cannot make a profit, then research and development will cease to exist, and COVID-19 will wipe out civilization. Conversely, PBMs invest zero dollars in research and development and are taking a wrecking ball to the very foundation on which the entire pharmaceutical industry was built centuries ago: the corner drugstore. Here is a QR code link to an interview with a PBM who specifically addresses and admits that the mission of her work is eliminating competition from the pharmacy business:

https://www.youtube.com/watch?v=LwosYxSkTAM

Since payers generally do not bring any pharmaceutical pricing knowledge to the table, they are vulnerable to price manipulations by the PBMs. Patients also have no clue, unless they happen to question the price difference, between using their insurance cards versus simply paying out of pocket.

Oftentimes, cash generic prices at the corner drugstore are cheaper than insurance-billed, PBM-mediated claims. That's a well-kept secret that PBMs go to great lengths to keep from being publicized, even going as far as contractually prohibiting pharmacists from potentially sharing cost-saving information with patients. Only recently are regulators and legislative bodies at the state level beginning to take notice and scrutinize these deceptive practices.

The president of the United States specifically mentioned that "our plan bans the Pharmacist Gag Rule, which punishes pharmacists for telling patients how to save money. This is a total rip-off, and we are ending it" (Trump, 2018). While there has been little federal follow up on this problem, many states are beginning to pass legislation to rein in the PBMs. Why then has the White House not intervened as promised?

As an educated consumer, make sure to always ask your pharmacist if you are getting the best price. Do not let the greedy PBM middlemen make you pay out the wazoo (OTW) for drugs that may only cost a few dollars if you circumvent the insurance card and simply pay cash. Also ask your pharmacist where your drugs were manufactured. Chances are that you will not be very happy with the answer.

The Organization for Economic Cooperation and Development (OECD) is an intergovernmental economic organization with thirty-seven member countries. Its mission is to stimulate economic progress and world trade. It is a forum of countries describing themselves as committed to democracy and the free market economy, providing a platform to compare policy experiences, seek answers to common problems, identify good practices, and coordinate domestic and international policies of its members (OECD, 2020). The United States spends the highest percentage of its gross domestic product (GDP) on health care expenditures among the nations of the world. The United States is also the only OECD nation that does not offer health care as a right (Bradley & Taylor, 2013; Niles, 2018). The United States ranks at the bottom of the industrialized world when it comes to health care, health outcomes, and overall life expectancy (OECD, 2019). Perhaps this is because we spend so much money on treatment of those who are already ill and allocate so few resources for prevention of acute and chronic disease. Additionally, many citizens cannot afford to purchase health insurance. While full-time salaried employees are typically offered some level of employer-sponsored health insurance, part-time workers and 1099 contractors are not usually offered health insurance. Health insurance is a major determinant of access to health care. Uninsured individuals cannot afford to utilize the expensive US health care system. Many patients with insurance have difficulty paying for their premiums, deductibles, and co-pays, as well as goods and services that their insurance does not cover. Employers are increasing the cost sharing of their employees for health care benefits and prescription drugs (Austvoll-Dahlgren et al., 2008).

As this book goes to press, we are simultaneously inundated by a tsunami of public health, national security, and economic disasters. The world is being overwhelmed by the opioid, diabetes, and COVID-19 pandemics. Inferior drugs (and, ironically, their lack of availability) from China and India are threatening our lives and our national security. Almost forty million workers filed unemployment claims during the first eight weeks of the coronavirus outbreak (*WSJ*, 2020). Large businesses like JCPenney and Neiman Marcus, as well as small businesses including gyms and yoga studios, hair salons, and restaurants, are being forced into bankruptcy due to the COVID-19 quarantines and shutdowns. Two percent of all small businesses and three percent of restaurants have already closed their doors permanently. "Analysts warn this is only the beginning of the worst wave of small-business bankruptcies and closures since the Great Depression" (Long, 2020). Unaffordable pharmacy co-pays continue to make it impossible for patients to afford to take their prescription medications as prescribed. If these were individual events occurring consecutively, we could more easily divide and conquer. Unluckily, the situation is much more ominous because all of the phenomena described above are happening simultaneously. Our country, along with the rest of the world, is beginning to reopen—cautiously in some locations and hastily in others. It remains to be seen if additional waves of COVID-19 will strike. The know-how of Big Pharma is shining through in the research and development of vaccinations and drugs to prevent, treat, and cure COVID-19.

Health Care Roulette is based on real news, not fake news. But anything stated in this book that is not specifically substantiated by a cited reference should be considered solely the author's opinion. The author wants you, the reader, to form your own conclusions by following the links to many published references provided via QR code and URL.

INTRODUCTION

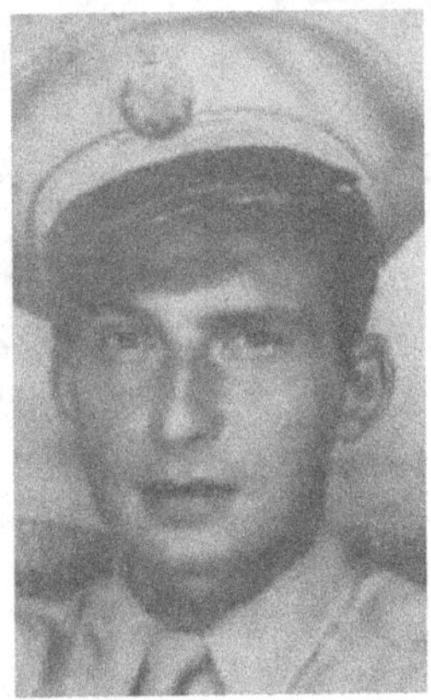

Private First Class George Tammara

World War II

In my opinion, June 6, 1944 is the single most important date in history. On that day, Operation Neptune, the largest sea-born invasion in history and part of the larger Operation Overlord, commenced as the Greatest Generation stormed the beaches of Normandy, France.

Our fathers, grandfathers, and great-grandfathers, along with our English and Canadian allies, braved annihilating machine-gun fire from the cliffs above the beaches. They courageously fought their way off the beaches, scaling the massive cliffs of Pointe du Hoc, and charged relentlessly to victory across France, Belgium, and Germany.

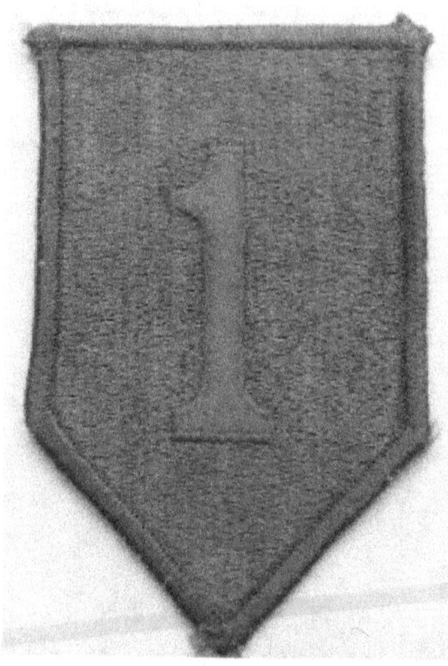

My grandfather, Private First Class (PFC) George Tammara, fought his way across Europe as an infantryman with the First Division ("the Big Red One"). He spent Christmas Eve of 1944 in Belgium, in a foxhole, fighting what was to become forever known as the Battle of the Bulge. He fought next in the Battle of Remagen, supporting the Ninth Armored Division and capturing the Ludendorff Bridge. This very battle was immortalized in the movie *The Bridge at Remagen*, starring George Segal, Robert Vaughn, and Ben Gazzara. On March 26, 1945, PFC George Tammara took an enemy bullet, and on March 28 he died a hero, just a few weeks before the end of the war. Victory in Europe was proclaimed on May 8, 1945. If not for the courage of the Greatest Generation, I would not be here today to write this book; nor would you be here to read it.

After the war was won, the European Recovery Plan, also known as the Marshall Plan, was implemented for the reconstruction of Western Europe. The United States invested billions of dollars into this recovery and rebuilding effort. In April of 1948, the Organization for European Economic Cooperation (OECC) was created. Headquartered at the Château de la Muette in Paris, the OEEC strived to establish a permanent organization to continue work on European recovery and to oversee the distribution of aid. The OEEC was the predecessor of today's Organization for Economic Cooperation and Development (OECD). The OECD is "an international organization that works to build better lives. Their goal is to shape policies that foster prosperity, equality, opportunity and well-being for all" (OECD.org).

Today, thanks in large part to the money that we poured in via the Marshall Plan, residents of England, Canada, France, Germany, and other industrialized nations, including our former enemies, enjoy good lives, complete with government-subsidized health insurance as a right of citizenship. Some countries have socialized medicine, some have privatized medicine, and some have a combination of both. The United States, on the other hand, has a patchwork of insurance plans that cost top dollar and provide skimpy coverage with astronomical out-of-pocket expenses, all the while shifting more of the cost burden to the patient. We will now compare and contrast a representative sampling of several health care systems, including the United States and some of our European counterparts.

Life Expectancy

Life expectancy is the key indicator of the overall health and well-being of a population. Public health experts and economists consider life expectancy as an important component of the measure of a nation's prosperity. Infant mortality rates and health risk behaviors are additional indicators that are used to evaluate the health status of a population. One might mistakenly assume that the United States would rank as superior to all other nations when it comes to life expectancy and other health indicators. After all, we spend significantly more money per capita on health care than any other nation. Certainly, our life expectancy rates should be much higher than they are (OECD, 2015).

The US average life expectancy was 78.8 years when I first started writing this book (Niles, 2018). The average life expectancy among the thirty-four member countries of the OECD is 80.5 years. Life expectancy in Japan is 84.1 years (Niles, 2018). Switzerland enjoys a life expectancy of 83.8 years. Mexico, with a life expectancy of less than seventy-five years old, is the lowest (Niles, 2018).

The United States' life expectancy has since decreased to 78.6 years as this book nears publication. Despite our enormous health care expenditures, our life spans are falling even shorter than the OECD average, ranking a dismal twenty-ninth (Niles, 2018). For the first time in years, life expectancy in the United States has actually decreased. We are seeing an increase in the overall mortality rate in the United States, causing a concerning decline in overall US life expectancy at birth (World Data Bank, n.d.). Among the explanations for the decrease in US life expectancy are the opioid epidemic and suicide, as well as unintentional deaths from drugs like fentanyl, heroin, and oxycodone. Our younger generations, as well as middle-aged adults, have alarming rates of depression and addiction. The United States has lost three-tenths of a year in life expectancy since 2014, an embarrassment for the country that saved the world from tyranny in World War II.

Deaths from influenza and pneumonia, particularly in the elderly and underserved populations without access to quality health care, have also contributed to the decline in US life span. Racial disparities in disease and death rates continue to be a problem. Tragically, as this book goes to publication, the COVID-19 pandemic has already killed hundreds of thousands of innocent souls and brave first responders across the globe, with the numbers rising every hour. Obesity and diabetes are two deadly epidemics that drive each other and take a huge cumulative toll on quality and quantity of life, inflicting significant morbidity and mortality, much of which is actually preventable. Those with diabetes and other comorbid conditions are also significantly more susceptible to the complications of COVID-19. The decrease in the US life span was driven by increases in the eight leading causes of death. Deaths from heart disease and stroke were up after declining for years. The trend is due to a combination of factors, with obesity and diabetes epidemics being significant contributors.

It remains to be seen how epidemiologists will calculate the devastating effects of COVID-19 into the life span equation for upcoming years. That determination is likely to be complex, as variables such as diabetes and comorbid conditions including heart disease and chronic bronchitis or emphysema (COPD), along with the social determinants of health (zip code, race, ethnicity, education, employment, income, and access to healthy foods and quality health care) are significant contributors to health outcomes and life span (ADA, 2020; CDC, 2017). For example, African Americans and Latinos are routinely subject to health disparities and may not be able to afford to take their medications as prescribed due to cost (Shenolikar et al., 2006).

Medication nonadherence has been proven to have negative physical outcomes on morbidity (disability) and mortality (death and life span). As we factor in diabetes, heart disease, COPD, and now COVID-19, we are seeing a disproportionate number of deaths in populations that were already at higher risk for poor health outcomes. When it comes to COVID-19, we are *all* at risk. The public health construct of *social justice* comes into effect when certain demographic groups are more at risk than others. Urban areas, because of population density, are where the virus emerged the fastest. Social justice is based on the premise of human rights and equality and can be defined as "the way in which human rights are manifested in the everyday lives of people at every level of society" (Cefalu et al., 2018; Conrad, 2007, Diclemente et al., 2013; Gourzoulidis et al., 2017; Henk et al., 2018; Pawasakar et al., 2018). Persons living in poverty are more likely to be in poor health and less likely to use the health care system compared to those with higher incomes. An uninsured person, for example, might avoid the expense of seeing a primary care provider for a particular ailment (chest cough, for example) that could be easily resolved with a short course of medication. By the time the same uninsured patient finally seeks care in the emergency department, he or she has already progressed to a more severe diagnosis (pneumonia, for example) that is associated with an increased risk for morbidity and mortality and is more expensive to treat (Diclemente et al.).

Continuing on the topic of life span, the increase in accidental deaths and suicides ties in directly with the opioid epidemic that is gripping our nation and is playing a role in the life expectancy decrease (Niles, 2018). Patients currently taking prescribed opioids for pain, individuals misusing illegally diverted prescription opioids, and those using illicit opioids such as heroin or fentanyl are at risk for unintentional opioid overdose. As such, health care practitioners, family and friends of people who have opioid-use disorders, and community members likely to come into contact with people at risk for opioid overdose can save lives if they know how to use Narcan (naloxone) and keep it within reach. Here are links to videos on how to use Narcan:

It is of critical importance for rescuers to call EMS or 911 even after a patient is revived with Narcan because the opioids have a longer duration of action (half-life) than the Narcan, and the revived individual is still at risk for falling back into respiratory arrest and death. In most situations, Good Samaritan laws will protect those who call EMS so that there is no risk of being accused or prosecuted for drug offenses.

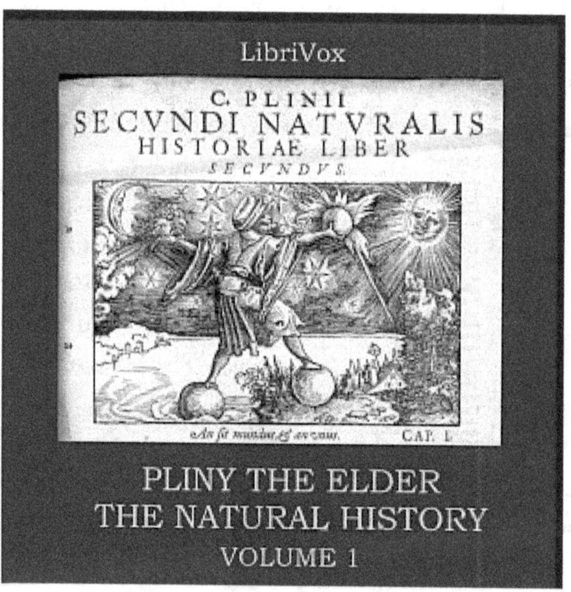

Pliny the Elder is very famous for his publication *The Natural History*, originally written in AD 77, which includes discussion of matters related to medicine. Specifically, Pliny speaks of plants that yield useful drugs. He discusses hundreds of drugs, including poppy and opium. Even as you are reading this, we are living through the worst modern-day opiate / narcotic-drug epidemic in history. Every day the headlines are full of stories about heroin overdoses in our communities. It's ironic that Pliny took notice, so long ago, that opium induces sleep and can be fatal. Pliny the Elder died a hero, before completing his work, in AD 79 while attempting to rescue his friends from the eruption of Mount Vesuvius. The remainder of his writings were published posthumously by his nephew, Pliny the Younger.

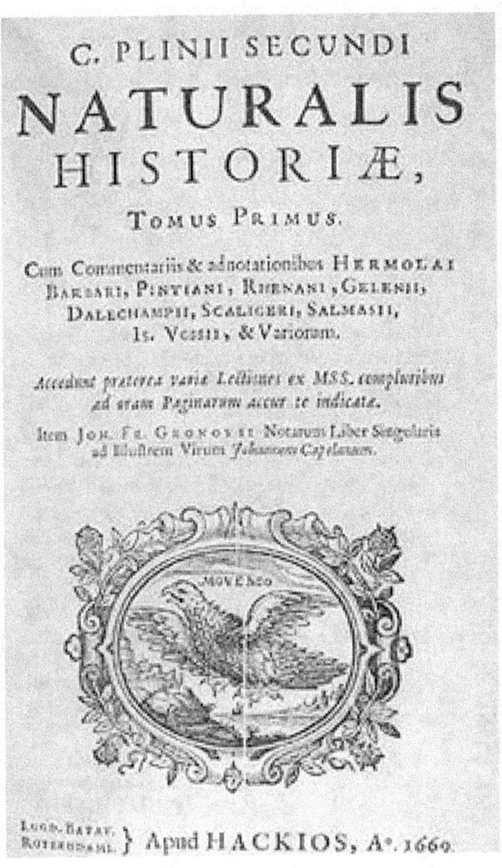

Life expectancy equals the average number of years a person born in a given country is expected to survive if mortality (death) rates at each age remain steady in the future. Most people live either much longer or much shorter lives than what the average life expectancy predicts. Low life expectancy is usually the result of very high child mortality rates. Those people who survive the dangers of childhood can expect to live to a relatively old age, even in countries with very low life expectancy. We will soon have more older people than children and more people at extreme old age than ever before.

As we age, quality of life becomes a very important indicator, one we must pay close attention to. There is always the danger of an expansion of morbidity, an increase in the prevalence of disability, as life expectancy increases. It's not only how long we live but also how well we can function into advanced age. The twin epidemics of obesity and diabetes are contributing factors to quality of life, morbidity, and mortality.

If not treated properly and monitored constantly, diabetes can lead to neuropathy, kidney disease, stroke, gastroparesis, and skin and eye complications. Once diagnosed, patients face difficulties in making lifestyle changes related to exercising, eating healthier foods, and managing stress. There are also challenges that must be overcome related to testing blood-glucose levels and taking daily pills and/or insulin injections.

The range of psychological, social, economic, and environmental factors that influence health status are known as *determinants of health*. Biological and genetic makeup, individual behaviors, social interactions, physical environment, and access to health care are all examples of determinants of health. Determinants of life expectancy include ongoing wars, epidemics and pandemics, acute and chronic diseases, and other determinants of health. Disparities in access to health care and healthy foods also play a role in life expectancy, as do the zip codes in which people reside.

It remains to be seen what effect the current coronavirus pandemic will have on life span. It is also unknown how many people will die from taking untested, dubious remedies for COVID-19. It is a perilous situation when government leaders *with good intentions* (but with no medical training) contradict trained medical professionals and epidemiologists. How many US governors, congresspersons, and cabinet officials have graduated from medical school? Pharmaceutical companies are racing to develop safe and effective drugs to prevent, treat, and cure COVID-19. We must be patient and rely on science and scientists to find these treatments. Politicians, witch doctors, shamans, and snake oil salesmen are not licensed to offer medical information. The World Health Organization (WHO) has published a list of guidelines to combat the dissemination of unreliable information. Readers are encouraged to rely on evidence-based data published by reputable scientific bodies such as the WHO, CDC, and FDA. For example, wearing masks, washing hands, and practicing social distancing appear to be helpful in mitigating the spread of the virus. So let's do that!

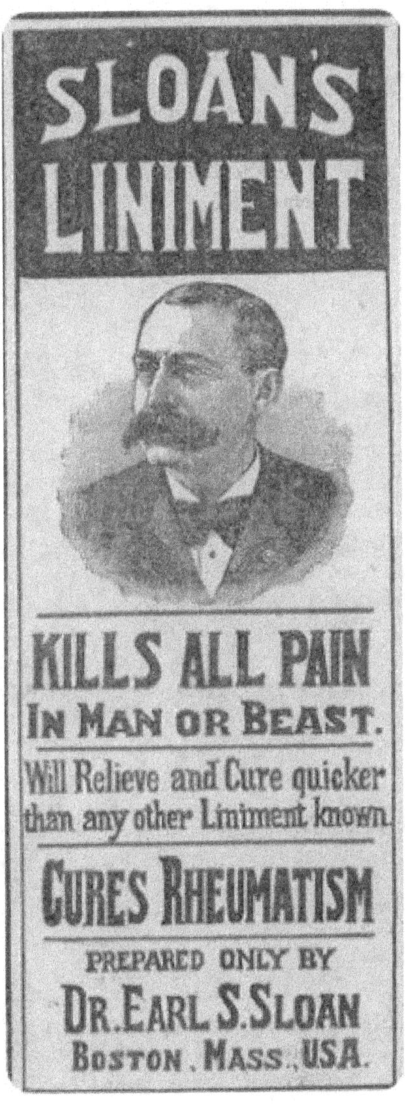

Advertisement from the patent medicine era

COMPARATIVE HEALTH CARE SYSTEMS

Organization for Economic Cooperation and Development (OECD)

The Organization for Economic Cooperation and Development (OECD) is the offspring of the OEEC and came into being in 1961 with a mission to develop and promote economic progress and stimulate world trade and social policies among its members. OECD member nations include Australia, Austria, Belgium, Canada, Chile, the Czech Republic, Denmark, Estonia, Finland, France, Germany, Greece, Hungary, Iceland, Ireland, Israel, Italy, Japan, Korea, Luxembourg, Mexico, the Netherlands, New Zealand, Norway, Poland, Slovak Republic, Slovenia, Spain, Sweden, Switzerland, Turkey, the United Kingdom, and the United States.

Canada

Geographically, Canada is the largest nation in North America. Governmentally, Canada is a constitutional monarchy. Citizens enjoy publicly funded comprehensive universal health care coverage with almost no out-of-pocket charges, although there are a few minor exceptions. The Canadian health care system is called Medicare and works similarly to our Medicare system, except that *everyone* is covered, not only senior citizens and the disabled. All insured residents are legally entitled to all covered health services provided by the health care plan on equal terms. A health card is provided via the local government to each citizen who enrolls in the program in each province. The federal government, in turn, provides health care funding to each province. Unlike the United States, where those with Blue Cross get the red carpet rolled out and those on Medicaid get the bum's rush, everyone in Canada receives the same level of care.

All essential basic care is covered, including maternity but not including mental health and home care. As we have seen in the United States, mental health coverage is extremely important, especially in light of the increasing incidence of natural disasters, violent attacks, and pandemics in recent years.

Basic services are provided by private physicians, who are all reimbursed by a single government payer. Unlike the United States, where a multitude of providers submit a tsunami of invoices to a hodgepodge of disorganized, unrelated payers, often via a network of for-profit middlemen who also extract fees, all providers in Canada are reimbursed by the government at the same rate. Similar to the United States, health care providers in Canada are mostly private. Canada utilizes a single-payer system where providers are paid publicly at government-negotiated fee-for-service rates. Providers have to accept the government's reimbursement and cannot "balance bill" the patient for the difference. Luxuries such as private hospital rooms, cosmetic surgery, and certain nonessential elective surgeries are not covered by the government but may be paid out of pocket or via private insurers. While prescription drugs, glasses, dental care, and long-term care are not covered by Medicare, most people have supplemental plans that do cover these goods and services as well as rehabilitation, home care, and private rooms in hospitals (Johnson et al., 2018).

Canada's universal health care system differs significantly from that of the United States, where upward of fifty million people are uninsured (Commonwealthfund.org, 2019). For those Americans with health insurance, coverage varies from skimpy to comprehensive. Paradoxically, those Americans with the "best" insurance often cannot afford to use their insurance due to insurers' shifting the cost burden from themselves to the patients (Austvoll-Dahlgren et al., 2008). In the United States, costs—including premiums, deductibles, and co-pays—are being systematically driven up by for-profit insurers and pharmacy benefit manager (PBM) behemoths who have hungry stockholders to satisfy. In Canada, insurance plans must be administered and operated on a nonprofit basis by a public authority, with no co-pays for medically necessary care. The United States has an incalculable array of insurance plans, with unpredictable variations in the level of coverage and costs that vary from one geographic area to another.

If you live in Philadelphia and need medical care in Florida or California, you might be forced to pay cash. If you change employers, it is likely that your health insurance will also be switched. Canadians can freely travel or relocate from one province or territory to the next with no worries about the continuity of their health coverage. Insured people must also be provided access to hospitals, doctors, and dentists in proximity to their residences, although transportation costs can still present a barrier to access for some (Johnson et al., 2018). On the downside, there are tremendously long wait times to see a specialist, for diagnostic testing (X-ray, MRI, etc.), and for certain medical procedures. You might just die waiting. Canada, however, doesn't have to deal with PBMs!

United Kingdom

The English health care system operates according to the Beveridge model of socialized medicine. Coverage is universal for all citizens of the United Kingdom through the National Health Service (NHS). The government is the single payer, funding all health care via taxes and providing free health care for all citizens as a public service. Unlike in the United States, where virtually nothing comes without a hefty price tag, everything from ambulance transport and emergency department visits to long hospitalizations, all types of surgeries, radiation, and chemotherapy are all included in the smorgasbord for "free" in England. There is a payroll tax that finances it all. Even so, there is a considerable backlog for surgical procedures, drugs are rationed, and emergency department waits can be extremely prolonged.

Citizens of England have similar access to primary care physicians (PCPs) compared to citizens of the United States. In fact, primary care providers are the gatekeepers, carefully evaluating each patient to determine who deserves a referral to see a specialist. Unlike in the United States, Canada, and France, where providers are private, the government employs and controls all providers in the United Kingdom. Relatively few people in the United States can afford long-term-care insurance.

When Americans get chronically ill, we are forced to spend down all our resources and then apply for Medicaid (welfare). We subsequently get whisked off to substandard nursing homes that are too heavily dependent on Medicaid to provide high-quality care. Due largely to the high proportion of Medicaid patients, US nursing homes, as we have witnessed during the COVID-19 pandemic, are essentially giant petri dishes and are not where we want to spend the rest of our lives. In England, long-term care is a right of citizenship that is automatically provided by the government, with no out-of-pocket expenses to worry about. Unlike the United States, the English are not demoted from middle class to the poverty level as a condition to being entitled to long-term care.

In a situation similar to that of Canadians, the English have longer wait times to see specialists and less access to technology for diagnostic testing. The English are not always happy with their health care system and there have been protest marches on occasion, but at least it's free. Even with all of the high-tech diagnostics available in the United States and the better access (only if you can afford it) to health care, both the United States and England have one thing in common: too many preventable deaths (Johnson et al., 2018). We all need to focus more on public health! England, like the rest of the world (except for the United States), does not have to deal with PBMs!

Germany

The Germans utilize the Bismarck model of health care. Germans have cost-sharing responsibilities (via payroll deduction) and utilize private providers and payers (Reid, 2010). In Germany, "sickness funds" are legally required to provide a comprehensive set of benefits. Sickness funds are private nonprofit insurance companies that collect premiums from employers and employees. These include physician ambulatory care provided by physicians in private practice, hospital care, nursing home care, a wide range of preventive services, and even visits to health spas. Unlike the United States, patient cost sharing is minimal. The funds, similar to disability insurance, also provide additional cash payments to those who are unemployed as a result of illness (Johnson et al., 2018). Germany does not have to deal with PBMs!

France

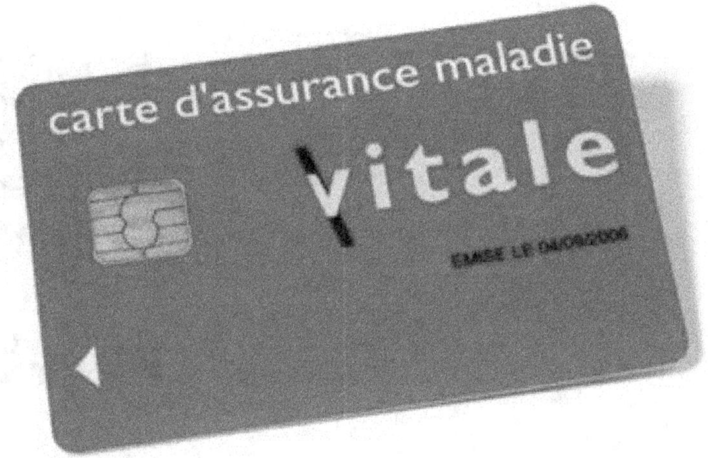

The French have payroll taxes that fund a large part of health care spending, and they actually spend significant money (11.6 percent of GDP) on health care. Unlike the United States, where insurance premiums are often astronomical, the French government dictates what percentage of an employee's salary will be deducted toward health insurance premiums. Since deductions are based on a percentage of income, most citizens can afford their premiums. Unlike the United States and the United Kingdom, France has some of the very best health outcomes of all OECD countries ("The Health Care System of France," 2018). A French citizen simply shows a *carte vitale* (card of life), and all services are covered and recorded digitally. Co-pays exist, but they are reimbursed later by the government (Reid, 2010). France does not have to deal with PBMs!

The U.S. has the lowest life expectancy at birth among comparable countries

Life expectancy at birth in years, 2016 or nearest year

Country	Years
Japan	84.1
Switzerland	83.7
Australia	82.5
Sweden	82.4
France	82.4
Comparable Country Average	82.2
Canada	81.9
Austria	81.7
Netherlands	81.6
Belgium	81.5
United Kingdom	81.2
Germany	81.1
United States	78.6

Notes: Data for Canada & France are for 2015.

Source: Kaiser Family Foundation analysis of 2018 OECD data: "OECD Health Data: Health status: Health status indicators", OECD Health Statistics (database) (Accessed on January 25, 2019).
• Get the data • PNG

Peterson-Kaiser
Health System Tracker

THE US HEALTH CARE SYSTEM: HOW DO WE COMPARE?

Even though we saved the world from tyranny and then spent countless billions to rebuild it, we are not entitled to the same health care coverage rights as our allies. In other words, even though the United States is the richest and historically the most magnanimous nation, we do not have universal health coverage for our own citizens. Harry S. Truman did promote universal health care in his Fair Deal of 1949, but it was defeated by the opposition.

World War II served as the stimulus for the beginning of employer-sponsored insurance in the United States. During World War II, the government passed the Stabilization Act, designed to limit employers' freedom to raise wages based on competition for scarce workers. While the act required that wages stay level, employers were permitted to provide health benefits (worth not more than 5 percent of the employee's income). Health benefits became an incentive to attract good workers. Additionally, beginning in 1954, the health benefits were not considered taxable, making them even more valuable to both employees and employers. Workers did not have to pay income tax or payroll tax on those benefits.

With nationwide quarantines associated with COVID-19 causing widespread economic devastation, much of the workforce has become newly unemployed and, therefore, uninsured. This is concerning because it has been established that those without health insurance are more likely to not be able to take their medications as prescribed due to cost (Gourzoulidis et al., 2017; Pawasakar et al., 2018; Shah, 2019). Thanks to the $700 billion government stimulus via the Paycheck Protection Program loans and grants, many small businesses will hopefully spring back to life as the environmental situation resolves. Nonetheless, the *Washington Post* has reported that more than one hundred thousand small businesses have already been forced to throw in the towel due to the virus (Long, 2020).

Financial Burden of High Out-of-Pocket Drug Costs in the United States

In the United States today, the cost burden of employee insurance is shared by the employer and the employee. Employees typically have certain out-of-pocket responsibilities such as premiums, deductibles, and co-pays.

Employed people with "good insurance" may still have very large out-of-pocket expenses. In the United States, costs, including premiums, deductibles, and co-pays, are driven up by for-profit insurers who have hungry stockholders to satisfy. As the *Columbus Dispatch* recently reported, Ohio fired a pharmacy benefit manager (PBM) for violating its contract by failing to pass along drug price savings while pocketing the money instead. Ohio attorney general Yost was quoted as saying, "They took our money," as he vowed to take action against PBM middlemen (Schladen, 2020).

https://www.dispatch.com/news/20190219/
yost-promises-more-action-against-pharmacy-middlemen-they-took-our-money

Meanwhile, federal antitrust regulators foolishly continue to approve the vertical integration between insurers, PBMs, and chain pharmacy providers. As these consolidations materialize among and between health care entities, consumers are left with little freedom to choose their own medical providers and absolutely no freedom to choose their own provider pharmacies. It is inconceivable that while horizontal mergers and acquisitions are blocked by the Department of Justice, vertical consolidations are not deemed to be antitrust. Scan below to observe actual data showing how patients are struggling to afford their prescription drugs (University of Minnesota, 2016).

http://statehealthcompare.shadac.org/map/73/percent-who-made-changes-to-medical-drugs-because-of-cost-in-the-past-year-by-age#13/15/110

This book is absolutely not anti—chain pharmacy or anti—mail-order pharmacy. It is about patients' *freedom to choose* the providers they wish to patronize. It's totally acceptable to offer patients the option of choosing to utilize chain pharmacies or mail-order pharmacy. All the same, there has to be a level playing field, with identical terms (co-pays and days' supply) offered to all patients across all providers—and the same level of reimbursement provided transparently to all providers.

With less pharmacy competition and fewer choices for consumers, the quality of health care is already declining. With the traditional corner drugstore on the verge of extinction, the supersized chain and mail-order pharmacies will soon have a captive audience. By systematically targeting and eliminating competition in the drug business, the health care system provides more limited access to drugs and increases price gouging. Senior citizens and underserved populations that depend on free same-day delivery service from small community pharmacies are suffering the most.

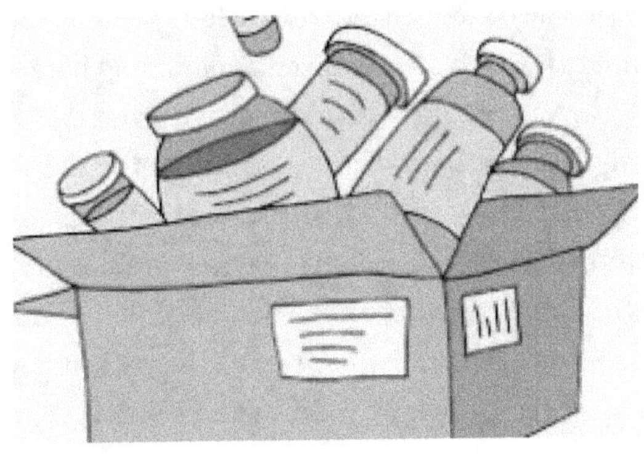

While mail-order pharmacies boast that they save money for the health care system, they actually create millions of dollars of unused, wasted drugs by automatically shipping large quantities of unwanted products. Here is a video proving that automatic mail-order shipments represent a huge waste of money, not a cost-saving measure as touted by the PBMs that own them and make windfall profits from them.

Traditional Medicine and Public Health

We as a society have, at many levels, become complacent with the role of medical care in our health care system. An army of doctors, assisted in large part by residents, interns, physician assistants, nurses, and other team members, diagnose and treat our individual health problems. Our health care system is like a revolving turnstile at a busy subway station with thousands of nameless, faceless commuters coming and going.

While many people have access to health care, not everyone has true access. Some patients get lost in the shuffle and never actually receive the health care that they need. Health care providers are under pressure and in a hurry to get to the next patient. As a consequence, all we often get is a quick blood pressure check and an abrupt dismissal. Hospitalized and nursing home patients are even less likely to have the opportunity to interact with their provider, with many physicians rounding early in the morning or late in the evening when patients are sound asleep. With the rise of the hospitalist physician, most patients do not even interact with their family doctors while they are hospitalized. The lack of communication with family doctors can be detrimental to the continuity of care. The family doctor is kept out of the loop until the patient gets discharged and eventually shows up at the primary care provider's office.

In many instances, by the time patients are properly diagnosed, their diseases or conditions are already at advanced stages. A prime example of this is type 2 diabetes, a highly preventable disease that has become a public health pandemic and a burden on health care systems globally.

There's a Pill for That

Traditional medicine and public health share the common goals of decreasing morbidity (sickness) and mortality (death) and increasing quality of life. They just approach them differently. Traditional medicine is reactive in nature and relies on traditional measures. A patient presents to the physician, and the physician instinctively whips out the prescription pad. Public health, on the other hand, is preventive in nature and uses a holistic approach.

Medicine deals with health from an individualized, retrospective approach, putting a Band-Aid on a preexisting wound and trying to minimize collateral damage. If a patient gets type 2 diabetes, for example, the doctor simply writes a prescription for metformin. If a patient gets COPD, the doctor writes a script for a bronchodilator inhaler.

Certainly, we are to be thankful that we do have these medications available. Yet perhaps we can prevent or delay the onset of disease. Public health looks at entire populations in a prospective, preventative framework in an attempt to achieve a healthy population. Public health strives to educate us on healthy eating and exercise so we don't get type 2 diabetes in the first place. Public health wants us to quit smoking (or not smoke in the first place) to avoid lung cancer and chronic obstructive pulmonary disease.

Of course, the family doctor will do his or her best to offer advice on weight loss or smoking cessation. Even so, by the time we arrive at the office or, more commonly, the urgent care center or the emergency room, we are already exhibiting symptoms. We are already sick, and we are there to be treated as quickly as possible and sent home.

Public Health

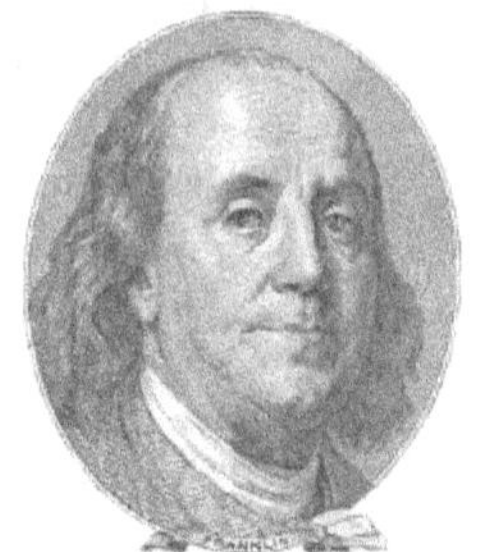

"An ounce of prevention is worth a pound of cure."
Benjamin Franklin

Public health deals with preventing disease and promoting health at the community or population level. While doctors treat us when we are sick, public health professionals try to prevent us from getting sick in the first place. While in medicine the patient is the individual person, in public health the patient is the community at large.

Doctors often integrate public health into their practices to some extent. For example, physician-initiated smoking-cessation programs save many patients from getting lung cancer. Still, the primary goal of traditional medicine is to provide treatment and medical care for those who are already suffering from a sudden ailment or a previously diagnosed chronic disease. There are so many acutely sick individuals who need immediate attention that it is difficult for primary care practitioners, emergency rooms, and urgent care centers to focus on anything other than acute care—prevention thus becomes unlikely.

With the fee-for-service system, physicians previously had the autonomy to practice medicine and take care of their patients as they saw fit. Sadly, doctors (and other providers) have evolved into puppets of the insurance companies and managed-care organizations. Physicians only have approximately fifteen minutes to spend with each patient from start to finish, including clerical duties such as record entry. Through not due to any fault of their own, there is little, if any, time left over for primary or secondary prevention. It is quicker and easier to remind the patient to lose weight, write a prescription for a statin, and move on to the next patient. It's not that doctors don't want to spend more time with their patients; it's that managed care does not permit them to. Insurance companies should allocate thirty minutes to physicians to properly examine each patient, ask and answer medical questions, and engage in programs to promote health and prevent disease.

Today, managed care has forced many private physicians to sell their practices and retire if they can afford to. Otherwise they become salaried employees of the health care organizations that acquire their practices. Physicians often lose their autonomy and have to see a certain number of patients per day while following specific formularies that limit their abilities to make effective therapeutic choices in the best interests of their patients.

Public health professionals exist with the mission of decreasing morbidity (sickness) and mortality (death) and are employed full time with the sole purpose of spreading knowledge of the benefits of preventative measures. These measures include handwashing to reduce the transmission of germs, immunizations to prevent influenza and pneumonia, healthy diets to prevent obesity and type 2 diabetes, and exercise to promote cardiovascular health.

Public health is the "ounce of prevention," and traditional allopathic medicine is the "pound of cure." The interdependence between public health and traditional medicine is very strong yet often overlooked. Our personal medical, physiological, and psychological health outcomes ultimately depend on the environments in which we live and work, as well as a vast array of modifiable and nonmodifiable risk factors and determinants. Public health takes a holistic approach, focusing on physical, mental, spiritual, and emotional well-being. Holistic medicine includes complementary alternative medicine (CAM) therapies such as yoga, meditation, tai chi, reiki, art therapy, and music.

When it comes to preventing acute and chronic diseases, we have little control over nonmodifiable risk factors such as age, ethnicity, and family history. Conversely, many of the modifiable risk factors such as smoking cessation, healthy diet, and regular exercise are targetable by public health interventions. Smoking-prevention and smoking-cessation programs, for example, can help reduce the occurrence of many diseases including cancer, emphysema, and chronic bronchitis. But we have had drastic underinvestment in public health and prevention while we simultaneously spend astronomical amounts on treating those who are already ill (Himmelstein & Woolhandler, 2016).

Health care policy is an important driver of quality of care provided and quality of life that results from the care provided. This includes not only the treatment of existing conditions in those who are already sick but also the prevention of illness in those who are still relatively healthy. For example, by promoting smoking cessation and vaccinations, we can reduce morbidity (sickness and disability) and mortality (death) associated with diseases such as cancer, COPD, influenza, and pneumonia.

Although the United States does not lead the world in longevity, the world is living longer due to advances in medicine, vaccinations, and preventive health. Acute pandemics from long ago like the plague, cholera, typhoid, smallpox, the Spanish flu of 1918, and now the lethal COVID-19 take their toll quickly and strike fear into all of us. As this book is being written, hundreds of thousands are dying of a pandemic reminiscent of plagues from the Middle Ages. But millions more are also dying slowly of chronic pandemics such as diabetes, obesity, and HIV/AIDS—and individuals with these comorbid conditions are at an even higher risk of succumbing to COVID-19.

Nonmodifiable Risk Factors for Disease

Genetic factors, family history, and increasing age are examples of nonmodifiable risk factors for acquiring certain diseases and medical conditions. Advanced age, for example, is a strong predictor of mortality from most any acute illness or chronic disease.

We cannot change our family histories regarding sickness and health, and we may be at risk for the same medical conditions as previous generations. For example, type 2 diabetes has very strong genetic links that make those with family histories more susceptible to it. Other nonmodifiable risk factors for type 2 diabetes include ethnicity, with Native Americans, Latinos, and African Americans being at higher risk for type 2 diabetes than Caucasians. Increasing age is a risk factor for incidence, prevalence, morbidity, and mortality in most chronic diseases, including diabetes. For example, as we age, our risk of acquiring type 2 diabetes increases, as does our risk of developing complications from the disease and dying from or with the disease.

This all makes sense if we think about it because we are not immortal. Eventually, we are all going to die from something. Therefore, if we are fortunate enough to avoid falling victim to the risks associated with childhood, it is likely that we will have a good shot at living longer and dying slowly with one or more chronic diseases. Very often, the disease will not even kill us; we will die *with* that illness but not *from* it.

Modifiable Risk Factors for Disease: Environmental Health

While there are some risks that we cannot change, many environmental factors in the community can be identified, acknowledged, and modified. Environmental regulations can and have been implemented and enforced. The prescription drugs in our medicine cabinets are very likely being used to treat illnesses or diseases that were triggered by environmental exposure.

For example, type 2 diabetes has many modifiable risk factors, particularly obesity. Obesity and type 2 diabetes are considered to be twin epidemics that feed upon each other. Early men were hunters and gatherers, foraging for their meals and burning calories as they did so. Today, we simply pull up to the fast-food window and load up on saturated fat and carbohydrates. McDonald's alone spends more money on advertising than all the fruit, vegetable, milk, and dairy distributors combined. Sometimes we can make healthier choices, but often fast food and corner convenience stores are all that are nearby, leaving no healthy food options. The closest full-service supermarket is often a bus ride away.

Abraham Maslow's Hierarchy of Needs

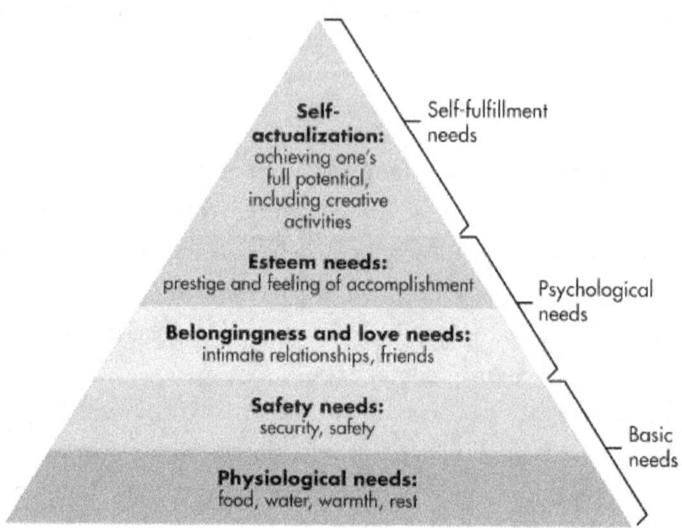

Abraham Maslow devised a motivational theory for psychology. This theory, also known as Maslow's hierarchy of needs, states that people strive to meet their needs in the form of a hierarchy. These needs are typically displayed in a pyramid, with the most basic needs being placed at the bottom.

Physiological needs are biological needs and must be met first for human survival. These are tangible survival requirements that include air, food, water, shelter, clothing, warmth, and sleep. If these most basic needs are not met, all the other levels of the pyramid become threatened. It follows, then, that when we are hungry we will eat whatever is available because we cannot survive otherwise (Maslow, 1943).

Primary literature has established direct relationships between living in areas considered food deserts—and the corresponding lack of access to healthy foods—and incidence and prevalence of type 2 diabetes. A food desert may be defined as an area within one mile of one's residence that does not have walkable access to a full-service supermarket or farmers' markets offering fresh fruits, vegetables, dairy products, poultry, fish, and meat. Diabetes runs higher in certain ethnic groups for genetic reasons but also for certain environmental reasons, including lack of access to healthy choices.

ACCESS TO HEALTH CARE

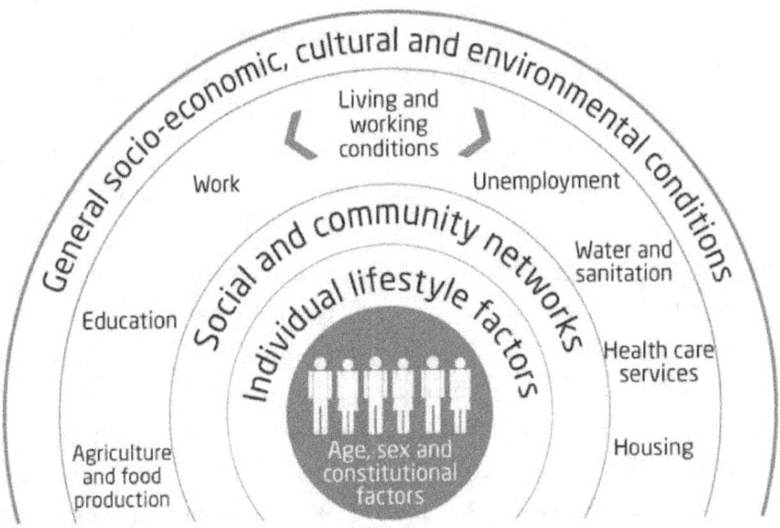

To paraphrase Bernie Sanders, "The richest have full access, and the poorest have almost no access" (Sanders, 2017). Disparities exist in access to health care, as defined by the social determinants of health, including race, ethnicity, socioeconomic status, age, sex, disability status, sexual orientation, gender identity, and residential location right down to the zip code. Disadvantaged individuals are often marginalized or discriminated against and will ultimately incur increased complications, higher treatment costs, and more frequent hospitalizations.

Diabetes is a prime example of how social determinants play a critical role in outcomes. Persons living in zip codes associated with food deserts often have no vehicle ownership or vehicle access and live far away (for example, more than a mile) from full-service grocery stores and supermarkets. This drives the obesity epidemic because disadvantaged populations are often forced to shop at corner mini-marts and convenience stores that are laden with highly processed foods of little nutritional value. The obesity epidemic, in turn, drives the type 2 diabetes epidemic, and vice versa. So begins the downward spiral that leads to heart disease, prediabetes, diabetes, and early death.

Barriers to health care mirror the social determinants of health and include the high cost of care, lack of adequate insurance coverage, lack of access to available services, lack of *true* access to available services, and cultural unawareness of health care providers. Take, for example, a Spanish-speaking patient who is assigned to a public health center provider who only speaks English. Due to a lack of multicultural staff at the health center, this patient is being denied true access, even though she is seeing a health care provider. Without a Spanish-speaking provider or interpreter, how will this patient have any clue how to follow the doctor's orders? What if the patient takes her medication improperly and has an adverse drug event?

As a result of the barriers to health care, there are innumerable individuals suffering with unmet medical and health needs. First off, there are those patients who never seek treatment or who delay treatment until a small problem has mushroomed into a full-blown emergency. As providers shift the cost burden to patients in order to combat moral hazard, emergency room co-pays can easily exceed hundreds of dollars, even for those with "good" insurance (Austvoll-Dahlgren et al., 2008). Once a sick individual finally decides to seek care, there are even more delays. How will the patient get to the hospital or clinic? Is there access to a personal vehicle, public transportation, or ride-sharing services such as Uber? Finally, upon arrival, how long will the patient have to wait to be seen by a provider? Does the provider speak the appropriate language, and/or is there an interpreter available (cultural sensitivity)? Are appropriate diagnostic tests performed (X-rays, CT scans, ultrasounds)? Are the patient's drug allergies noted, or will the emergency room prescribe penicillin to someone with a penicillin allergy? Is the patient insured? Uninsured patients are usually sicker, less likely to seek and receive adequate medical care or an accurate diagnosis, and more likely to have poorer health outcomes compared to patients that have health insurance. Additionally, those with no insurance are more likely to be unable to afford to take their medications as prescribed due to cost.

The preventive efforts of public health converge with traditional medicine, as primary care providers can offer screening services free of charge to their patients. The challenge for a primary care provider in preaching preventive measures is that managed care allows only so many minutes (approximately fifteen) per patient, and there is a never-ending stream of acutely ill patients who demand immediate attention (Bradley & Taylor, 2013). To again use diabetes as an example, primary prevention (education) can address the disease before it sets in. Secondary prevention can help those with prediabetes (the medicalized term for "borderline" or "a touch of the sugar") from progressing to diabetes (Conrad, 2007). Tertiary prevention can help persons with diabetes avoid microvascular complications (retinopathy, nephropathy, and neuropathy) that lead to blindness, end-stage renal disease, and amputations, as well as macrovascular complications (heart disease, circulatory problems) (Davidson,1981).

Zip Code versus Genetic Code

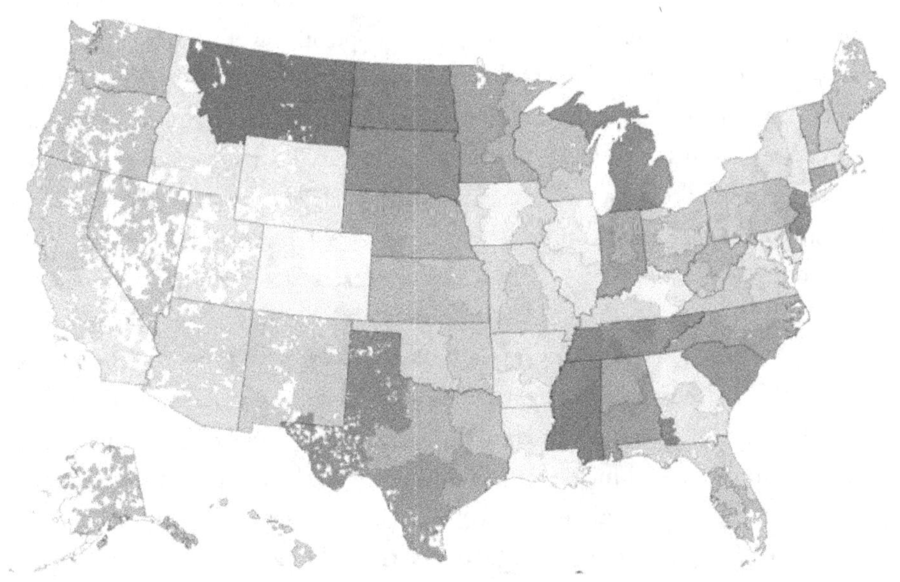

In order to gain an appreciation of the profound impact that our zip code has on our health outcomes, watch this video clip:

https://www.pbs.org/video/scetv-specials-zipcode-your-neighborhood-your-health-full-program/

Social determinants, including the environment and the conditions in which we work and live, weigh significantly in our risk of developing type 2 diabetes. Social indicators such as level of education, socioeconomic status (SES), and even the zip codes in which we reside play critical roles in determining the risk of developing type 2 diabetes, in coping with the complications, and in our overall longevity. This is concerning because many people of lower SES are affected by multiple social disparities that result in poor health outcomes (Bird et al., 2010).

For example, proper nutrition is of the utmost importance in the prevention and treatment of diabetes. Many individuals of lower SES reside in neighborhoods considered to be food deserts, devoid of healthy eating options. Corner grocery stores are notorious for stocking packaged junk food items with long shelf lives. These foods are loaded with refined carbohydrates that are energy dense and nutritionally empty. Residential segregation often prevents people from having access to supermarkets offering a wider variety of healthy choices such as nutritionally dense fruits and vegetables. Restricted access to healthy foods now places these lower-SES individuals at an even greater risk of developing type 2 diabetes and of succumbing to the complications of the disease (ADA, 2019).

These same individuals may also lack true access to adequate health care and qualified providers. For example, one of the individuals whom I interviewed made a very valid observation: "The doctor diagnoses diabetes, but the patient manages diabetes. The doctor sees the patient occasionally, but the patient must monitor their own blood sugar and follow their own diet and meal plan." Diabetes patients and/or their caregivers must be educated in many areas, including proper nutrition, regular exercise, and routine blood-glucose monitoring.

The diabetes epidemic is unequivocally connected to social determinants (e.g., access to jobs, health care, education, safe housing, language barriers, transportation, and healthy foods), social indicators (e.g., race, ethnicity, class, SES, education, and unemployment levels), and the health disparities that they produce (ADA, 2019). The COVID-19 pandemic is disproportionally taking aim at the very same populations, resulting in significant morbidity and mortality among African Americans, Latinos, and those residing in zip codes that are associated with disparities in access to health care.

The prevalence of diabetes both domestically and globally is approaching 10 percent, making diabetes not only an epidemic but also a pandemic (WHO, 2018). Diabetes monitoring at the individual level in the privacy of one's own home is accomplished with a personal glucose meter. These register spot values, providing a snapshot of an individual's blood sugar at any given point in time. Diabetes patients' skill sets at self-monitoring glucose are of critical importance to preventing complications in those already diagnosed with prediabetes or diabetes (secondary and tertiary prevention) since diabetes is the leading cause of blindness, end-stage renal disease, and amputation (ADA, 2019). On a broader scale, the hemoglobin A1C test, which is conducted by a physician at routine office visits, is usually monitored on a quarterly basis. Hemoglobin A1C is the gold standard in diabetes monitoring (ADA, 2019). As the average amount of glucose in the blood rises, the fraction of hemoglobin that becomes glycosylated increases proportionally. Higher HbA1c values are indicative of poorer control of blood-glucose levels. A rise in the hemoglobin A1C may indicate that the patient is in a state of prediabetes or perhaps is already diagnosable as having diabetes. The ADA dictates that an HbA1c value between 5.7 and 6.4 percent is indicative of prediabetes. An HbA1c of 6.5 percent or greater is diagnostic for diabetes. Hence, the HbA1c test is useful in preventive screenings as well as in quarterly monitoring of those already diagnosed. Significant differences exist between hemoglobin A1C reductions in patients with diabetes who filled their prescriptions as compared to patients who did not fill their prescriptions due to cost (Henk et al., 2018; Shah, 2008). This is important because hemoglobin A1C correlates with outcomes including morbidity (disability) and mortality (death).

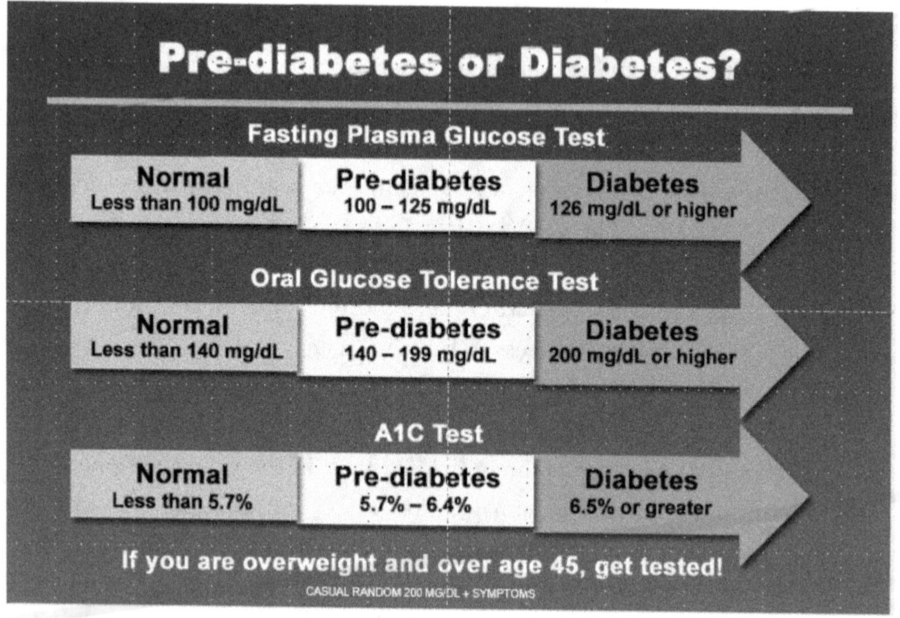

As it stands now, we have, at one end of the continuum, a nation notorious for disparities in access to health care for those who are uninsured or on Medicaid. Social determinants such as stress, discrimination, income, education, race, unemployment, housing, and even zip code come into play here, and these individuals often don't have access to quality health care. For example, the bum rush through the revolving door at the public health clinic does not necessarily represent true access.

At the other extreme, our working middle class has plenty of access for those who have insurance. Yet, due to perceived moral hazard, they are discouraged from utilizing health insurance by way of huge out-of-pocket expenses (premiums, deductibles, and co-pays). Moral hazard is the theory that reduced co-pays across the board (emergency rooms, specialists, prescriptions, etc.) lead to waste and an overall increase in prescription and medical costs by permitting patients to have access to more expensive services and medications for which the patients have less financial responsibility. The existence of moral hazard implies that more cost sharing will reduce the demand for health care services. While higher co-pays may keep hypochondriacs out of the emergency room, it will also prevent truly sick patients from seeking medical care when they need it most, leading to increased morbidity and mortality. While not "poor," this demographic group includes the author and the majority of people reading this book. We all know that it can be a financial hardship to use our coverage, even when we really need it. Insurance companies know this, too, and they do their very best to financially intimidate us from using our coverage, even though we already pay out the wazoo for our premiums, deductibles, and co-pays. *What good is having health insurance if you cannot afford to use it?*

Disability-adjusted life years (DALYs) are measures of disease burden (morbidity). The United States has the highest rate of disease burden among comparable countries. Contributing factors and areas that warrant our attention include the opioid epidemic, obesity, type 2 diabetes, and the current COVID-19 pandemic.

Understanding DALYs should allow those making health care policy to appreciate the vital role that primary prevention plays in overall quality of life, morbidity (DALY), and mortality. We live in a society where the vast majority of spending is focused on treating those already sick. Health care policy needs to allocate more resources toward prevention. Once disabled, individuals have few opportunities for benefiting from interventions that could save their lives. The Affordable Care Act (ACA) addresses this by including preventive care as an essential benefit. Primary prevention reduces DALYs.

Life expectancy in the United States, due in part to the opioid epidemic, has been leveling off compared to other OECD countries. Unlike chronic disease, which had, until the recent COVID-19 pandemic, largely replaced acute illnesses in terms of morbidity and mortality, the opioid crisis is reminiscent of pandemics from the past in which millions died acutely. The ACA acknowledges this by including treatments for substance abuse and mental health issues as essential health benefits.

The ACA requirement for food establishments to provide nutrition information is a major step in the right direction toward addressing obesity and type 2 diabetes issues. More than thirty million people with diabetes and more than ninety million with prediabetes contribute to the burden of chronic disease (DALY). The United States is in the midst of an obesity epidemic that is, in turn, driving a massive type 2 diabetes epidemic. Restaurant chains (many of which sell fast food) have shareholders to satisfy. Left unchecked, they will sell as much food as people are willing to buy, regardless of nutritional value (or lack thereof).

Rather than making a hasty choice to eat a high-calorie meal laden with saturated fat and cholesterol, an individual can now conduct an intelligent comparison between various menu offerings. He or she can then make an informed, educated decision as to which menu item to select. For example, a double-decker burger with fries may have over one thousand calories, whereas a grilled-chicken sandwich (especially if whole-grain bread is available) with no fries may have only a fraction of the calories. The individual can also decide not to patronize restaurants that do not offer healthy choices. As consumers get smarter by reading the gruesome details of what they are about to consume, they will realize that corporate greed and pleasing shareholders do not promote public health. Educated consumers (some, not all) will demand healthy choices and will probably be willing to pay a little more money for the opportunity to be healthy. Companies are stakeholders here, so it will be in their best interests to offer a wider array of healthier food options if they want to retain (and grow) their customer bases and keep their shareholders happy.

The social determinants of health care and the resulting disparities in access and true access play major roles in health outcomes and tie in with all the examples noted above. Education, including literacy and health literacy, ties in directly with primary prevention across all disease states. Eliminating food deserts and helping people learn to make smart nutritional choices would serve primary prevention roles in obesity and diabetes.

THE AGING POPULATION

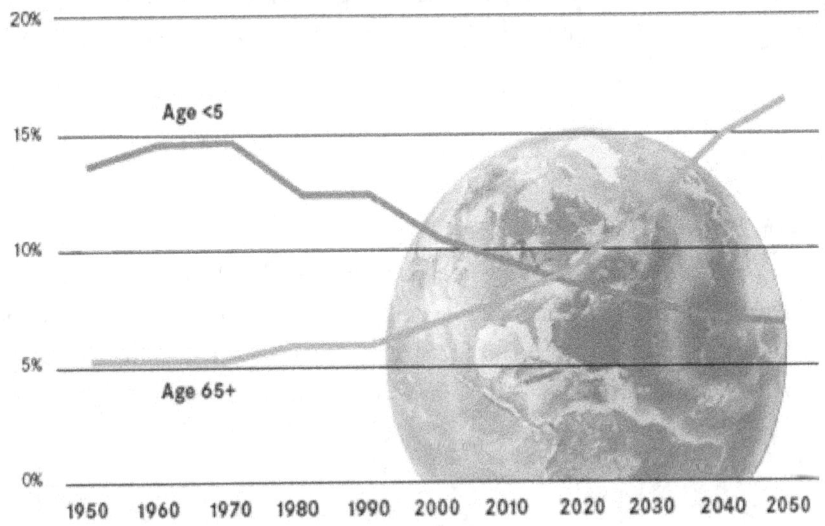

Source: *World Population Prospects: The 2010 Revision*, United Nations.
Adapted from *Global Health & Aging*, World Health Organization, 2011.

Patients, particularly the elderly and others on fixed incomes, often have to choose between purchasing their lifesaving prescription drugs and putting food on the table. The United States spends more money on prescription drugs than any other nation on planet Earth. As a population, the United States is growing older, and, as the following article emphasizes, this phenomenon is driving increases in health care expenditures:

https://www.pharmacytimes.com/publications/issue/2016/january2016/the-aging-popula-tion-the-increasing-effects-on-health care

Aging populations and the high cost of specialty drugs for diseases like cancer and hepatitis will continue to contribute to the increases in pharmaceutical spending. The rising cost burden of health care should not become a life sentence of poverty for those who are already struggling to survive (Garza, 2016; WHO, 2018).

We Are Living Longer

Prior to 1922, a diagnosis of type 1 diabetes was a death sentence. The discovery of insulin is only one example of how advances in scientific research and modern medicine have resulted in longer life spans. As we age, more chronic diseases will begin to manifest. This comes with the territory of longevity.

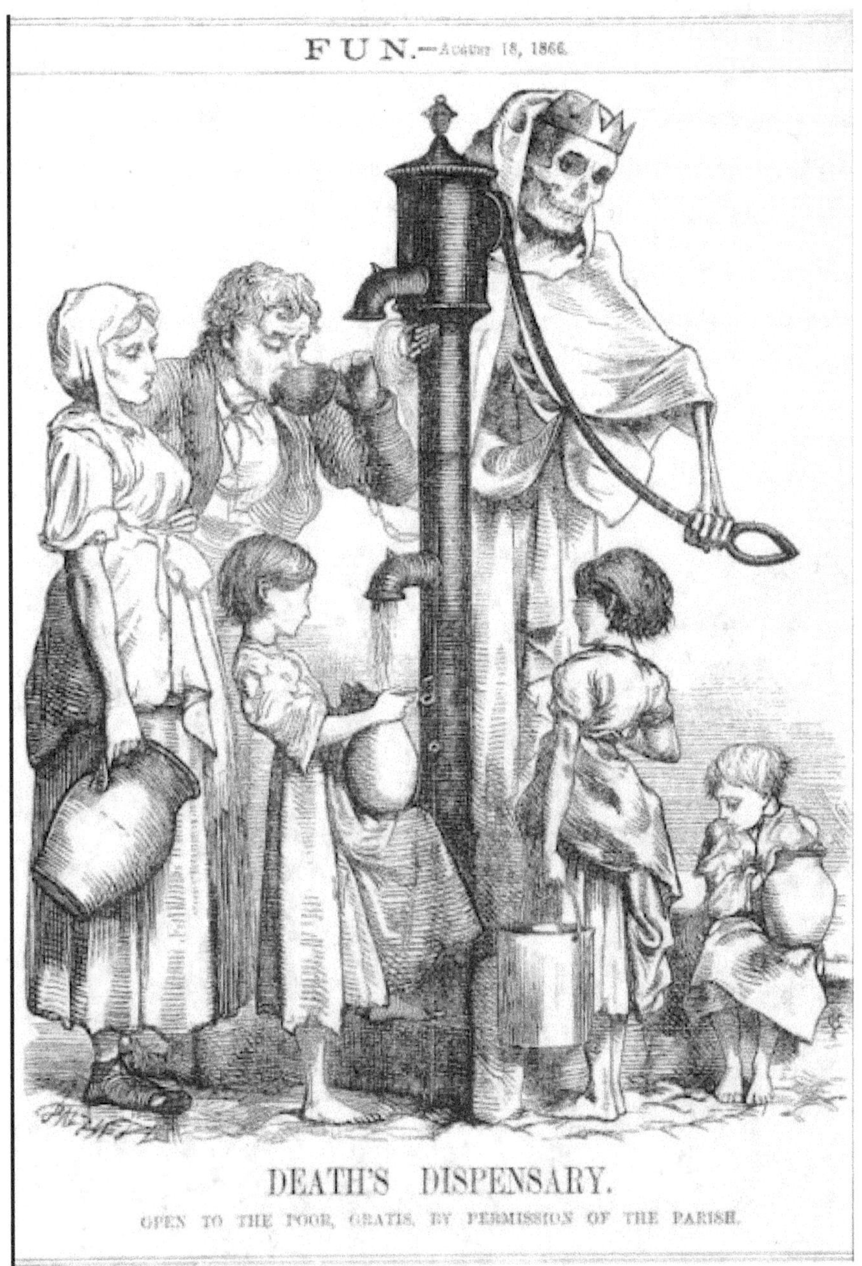

DEATH'S DISPENSARY.

OPEN TO THE POOR, GRATIS, BY PERMISSION OF THE PARISH.

In 1849 a cholera epidemic killed over fourteen thousand people in London. Up until 1854, when a second outbreak occurred in Soho, London, cholera was assumed to be an airborne disease. John Snow, an English physician, became a national hero because he was able to trace the contamination source to the city's water supply. Snow, by conducting house-to-house interviews of city residents, narrowed down the source of the sickness to a single water pump on Broad Street in Soho. He proved his point, that cholera is a waterborne disease, by having the local authorities remove the pump handle, effectively ending the cholera outbreak. "In 1854, the enterotoxic pathogen Vibrio cholerae was unknown. Nothing was known about the biology of the disease. Snow's conclusion that contaminated water was associated with cholera was based entirely on observational data" (Gordis, 2014, pp. 13–14). We do not necessarily need to know every detail of pathogenesis to be able to prevent disease. John Snow is considered the father of modern epidemiology, and his constructs are still being applied today to combat COVID-19.

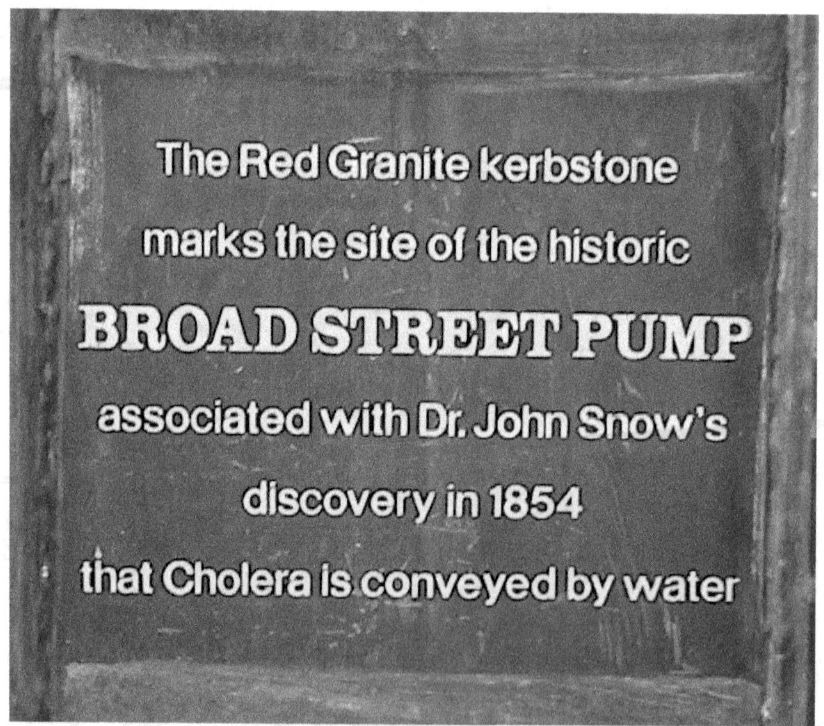

It's a spectacular accomplishment that we are no longer getting wiped out all at once by pandemics, as we were long ago (although the lethality of the current COVID-19 pandemic seems to indicate otherwise). We are not immortal; longer life expectancies indicate that we will die slowly from chronic diseases, and we will have the need for health care coverage and long-term care over the continuum of our life spans. Ischemic heart disease, cancer, asthma, emphysema, chronic bronchitis, and diabetes are going to get us eventually. With proper public health interventions for primary, secondary, and tertiary prevention, we may stand a better chance of dying *with* one or more chronic diseases than *from* them. *Now, in this COVID-19 environment, having our family doctor and our neighborhood pharmacist available is more important than ever before; it is paramount to our health care and our health outcomes.*

Dosing of medications in the elderly requires a specialized understanding of age-related changes in function and composition of the human body. As we grow older, all of our organs begin to deteriorate. The liver is typically responsible for the metabolism (breaking down) of the medications upon consumption by the patient. Our kidneys are in control of the excretion or clearance of the "used" drugs from the body. The elderly, by definition, have reduced capability to both metabolize and eliminate drugs from their bodies. It is important that health care providers assess liver and kidney function, adjusting doses accordingly. If drug doses are too high or the time interval between doses is too small, drugs will accumulate, causing a cascade of dangerous and potentially deadly consequences. Age-related changes in drug metabolism and excretion can result in exponential changes in magnitude of drug-related effects if drugs are not properly dosed. As a result, the elderly are often the unintentional victims of medication misadventures, including overdosage.

Hypertension (high blood pressure) is one of the most common ailments affecting the elderly. Otherwise normal doses of blood pressure pills, for example, can result in unexpected extreme drops in blood pressure called orthostasis. Some examples of blood pressure drugs that can cause orthostasis include alpha blockers, beta blockers, and other antihypertensives. In order to avoid orthostasis, patients should be instructed to arise slowly from lying or sitting positions, allowing time for their cardiovascular systems to equilibrate. Orthostasis causes countless numbers of falls, resulting in broken bones, hospital admissions, and deaths.

The elderly are also particularly sensitive to the oversedation associated with anxiolytics such as benzodiazepines (alprazolam, lorazepam, etc.) and sedative hypnotics (zolpidem, temazepam, etc.). When it comes to drug dosing in the elderly population, it is always best to start low and go slow. Start with the lowest-possible dose that is available, and gradually titrate upward to the minimum effective dose that produces the desired therapeutic outcome.

Long-Term Care

Long-term care is typically associated with the elderly. Additionally, there is a large population of individuals with physical and intellectual disabilities who depend on direct-care professionals for their day-to-day existences. While a typical skilled nursing or assisted living facility may be populated primarily by the elderly, personal care homes, boarding homes, and group homes that accommodate younger populations with special needs abound. These individuals with intellectual and developmental disabilities (IDD) require extra TLC to make sure that they receive the medical products and services to which they are entitled.

Many of the elderly are taking a dozen or more potentially dangerous medications prescribed by half a dozen different doctors who rarely, if ever, communicate with one another. Medication reconciliation is one intervention used to alleviate the risk of omissions, duplications of therapy, dosing errors, and drug interactions for those seniors who reside in long-term care environments. Medication reconciliation must occur when patients are discharged from the hospital and return back to the assisted living facility or nursing home. This is imperative in order to avoid polypharmacy because it's almost certain that some medications were discontinued during the hospital stay, while orders were likely written for new medications.

The Joint Commission mentions a five-step medication reconciliation process. First, the provider develops a comprehensive list of all the patient's current medications. Next, a list of all the medications to be prescribed is created. Now we compare the list of current medications to the new medication list, and we check for drug interactions and duplications of therapy. Clinical decisions as to what medications should be continued and discontinued are addressed at this point. In the last step, patients and caregivers are provided with information on the finalized medication regimen.

Without medication reconciliation, patients will be on a mishmash of old medications that were intended to be discontinued, plus all the newly prescribed medications. This is actually what happens every day in the lives of independent-living senior citizens who do not have access to senior-care consultant pharmacists.

In the long-term-care environment, senior-care (consultant) pharmacists provide a safety net to protect our fragile elderly population. Consultants play a critical role here, reviewing medical records and making recommendations to decrease doses of some medications and completely discontinue potentially dangerous medications.

For example, federal law requires routine attempts at the gradual dose reduction (GDR) of all psychotropic drugs in the elderly residing in nursing homes. *GDR* is a term used often in the long-term care setting. In the past, GDR has only been required for antipsychotic medications. Changes implemented in 2017 require GDR for all psychotropic medications. Antipsychotics, antidepressants, antianxiety medications, and sedative hypnotics are examples of broad categories of medications that now require GDR attempts. GDR involves the stepwise tapering of a dose to determine if symptoms, conditions, or risk can be managed by a lower dose.

Additionally, in order to minimize medication errors as well as to prevent intentional "chemical sedation" of the elderly in nursing homes, all medications must contain the indication for which each medication is being prescribed. Facilities that do not comply will receive violations known as "F tags" upon annual reviews by state authorities and the Joint Commission.

HOSPITALS AND HOSPITALISTS

Prior to the turn of the twentieth century, hospitals were looked down upon as places for the poor. Physicians used patients as guinea pigs from whom to learn and on whom to practice. At that time we began to observe improvements in medicine, including the use of anesthesia so people didn't have to bite down on sticks during surgery. The germ theory of disease came into being, and aseptic techniques were introduced to prevent infections. Now, with better health outcomes, the middle class and wealthy flocked to hospitals for elective procedures.

In 1946 the Hill-Burton Act established federal funding for the construction of new hospitals. In 1965 Medicare was signed into law by President Johnson. The elderly poor were now covered by insurance rather than being "charity" cases, so hospitals could make money. Today, hospitals have again become environments that we do not want to be exposed to for any longer than is absolutely necessary. The overuse of broad-spectrum antibiotics has contributed to antibiotic resistance and the development of superbugs that are resistant to all antibiotics. Nosocomial infections are acquired in the hospital and are becoming the norm once again. It is estimated (or underestimated) that one hundred thousand or more hospitalized US patients per year succumb to such hospital-acquired infections. Just like those old TV commercials for the Roach Motel, we check in, but we may not check out. For these reasons, most patients view outpatient services as the faster, cheaper, and safer alternative to overnight hospital stays.

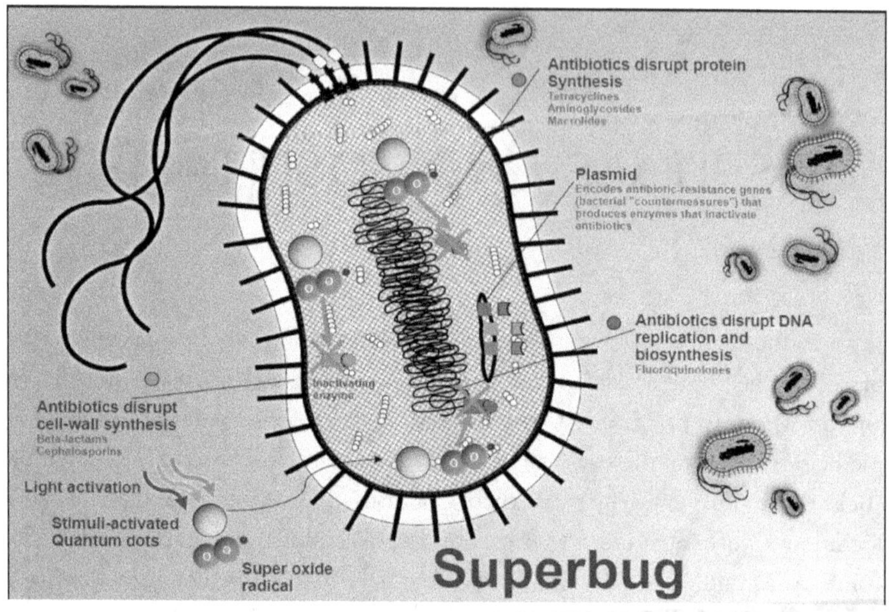

Gone are the days when family doctors rounded by their patients' bedsides each day when they were hospitalized. Today, it's the hospitalist (and not always the same hospitalist) who rounds each day. While these hospitalists are certainly capable and qualified physicians, they have probably never met the patient prior to admission and will never encounter the patient again postdischarge. This interruption of doctor-patient continuity of care across the inpatient and outpatient continuum is detrimental and can hinder the patient recovery process and even cause setbacks. Not only is continuity of care lost between the hospital and the family doctor, but there is also a lack of continuity of care within the hospital during the patient stay. How can the attending hospitalist look at you and determine if you appear better or worse than you did yesterday if he or she is not the same doctor who rounded yesterday or the previous day? All the hospitalist can do is peek at the chart or electronic medical record. You will not see the hospitalist(s) again after discharge, and your family doctor will have no clue what's going on until you follow up postdischarge. Physician work schedules are frequently made for the convenience of the prescriber, rather than being focused on patient-physician continuity. Patients are flipped to different attending hospitalists simply to lighten the workloads of the nursing and medical staff.

Hospitals are often staffed by "agency" nurses. So, in many instances, a patient may be seen by a different nurse every day, every shift: "This is my first day with this patient; I'll have to look at the chart." These nurses are competent, qualified, and compassionate. But they don't know the patients. Nurses should know their patients so that they can be in tune to any new signs or symptoms that might indicate relapse or improvement.

In at least one study, hospitalist discontinuity was associated with greater lengths of stays for certain diagnoses. Hospitalists may be conducting their obligatory patient rounds, but they are not contributing to the quality of life of these patients. When patients do not even have the opportunity to see the same providers they saw the previous day, there is no way for the providers to make clinical assessments to determine whether the patient is improving or getting worse (Nelson, 2015).

The hospitalist concept dates back to early European hospitals and is a step backward, creating a discontinuity in communication between patients, caregivers, family doctors, and other health providers. In the United States, there is limited access to and a lack of central databases for pertinent patient medical records. Competing for-profit providers are not always willing to share medical records with one another. Depending on whether the hospital discharge records arrive electronically, via snail mail, or not at all, your family doctor may or may not know your current drug regimen. Communication challenges among health systems and outpatient pharmacies frequently put patients in harm's way. Your pharmacy still has all your preadmission prescriptions and refills on file. So, when you get discharged from the hospital, you will end up taking all the new, postdischarge medications—and if you are not careful, you may also inadvertently take all the older medications that are still in your medicine cabinet.

This is where community pharmacists, if there are any of us left, play an indispensable role in medication reconciliation. The community pharmacist knows you and has complete electronic medication records of all your preadmission medications, which he or she can compare to your discharge orders. Allergies, drug interactions, and duplications of therapy can be flagged before any harm is done. Upon reviewing your hospital discharge orders, your corner druggist can tell you which of the medications on your kitchen table need to be continued and which need to be thrown away.

There are innumerable combinations of medication duplications and mis-adventures that occur post–hospital discharge. This is often called *polypharmacy* and can result in harmful drug interactions and readmission to the hospital. This is particularly concerning in the elderly, who by definition have compromised kidney and liver function and are therefore more susceptible to the toxic accumulation of drugs in the body. Additionally, this demographic group is constantly being admitted, discharged, and readmitted back and forth between hospitals and their independent living, assisted living, and nursing homes. This presents a recipe for disaster when multiple prescribers who never communicate with one another prescribe multiple medications for elderly patients they may never see again. The more drugs a patient takes, the higher the risk of overlapping side effects and adverse drug reactions (ADR).

POLYPHARMACY

Many elderly patients reside in long-term-care settings and are prescribed multiple overlapping drugs, providing duplicate therapy for the same indication. But the federally mandated monthly consultant pharmacist review acts as a safety net to flag and address these duplications of therapy that may not have been addressed by medication reconciliation. As drug regimens become increasingly more complex, these services are even more vital.

Unfortunately, there is no medication reconciliation in the community, so many patients are frequently subject to duplications of therapy, incorrect dosing regimens, and potentially fatal drug interactions. Polypharmacy is of particular concern when it comes to seniors since, by definition, they are more prone to potential adverse drug consequences. Again, seniors have medications in their possession from multiple prescribers who do not communicate with one another and have no clue what the others are prescribing. The more physicians an elderly person visits, the more drugs the patient is prescribed and the higher the risk for medication misadventures. This risk increases exponentially when the patient uses multiple pharmacies that do not share information with one another electronically. Their livers are not breaking down the drugs as fast, and their kidneys are not excreting the metabolites as efficiently as they did in their youths. Consequently, the half-lives of the drugs are increasing, and those drugs will accumulate in the elderly if not properly dosed for decreased liver and kidney function.

The more medical conditions an individual is diagnosed with, the more medications that individual is likely prescribed and the greater the risk of drug interactions and side effects due to polypharmacy. The elderly and, in particular, individuals with intellectual and developmental disabilities are more susceptible to medication misadventures than the general population. One thing to keep in mind is that when a drug is approved by FDA, it has been tested on only a relatively small number of people. It is not until later (post–marketing surveillance) that many of the side effects and drug interactions are discovered.

The practice of polypharmacy (having been prescribed multiple drugs from one or more classes of medications for one or more diagnoses, often resulting in duplication of therapy and unintended side effects) has been increasing in prevalence in the treatment of individuals with dual diagnosis (IDD and mental health disorder).

Individuals with intellectual disabilities have complex pharmaceutical care needs due to a high prevalence of multimorbidity. Patients may be seeing primary care providers as well as specialists in psychiatry, neurology, and others. It is likely that each practitioner is prescribing multiple medications for each individual. Polypharmacy results in a high prevalence of adverse drug reactions for those at risk.

In addition to following a healthy lifestyle and proper diet, medications are essential for managing the health-disease process. Prevention is key to not getting sick, while drug therapy is the main therapeutic resource to cure and control diseases. Safe medication use involves maintaining a balance of risks versus benefits while trying to avoid adverse drug events. Currently, the use of multiple medications is a problem, especially with the continuous introduction of new medications into the marketplace.

The worldwide epidemiological profile has been changing over the years. We are living longer, resulting in the population's aging and consequently in the predominance of noncommunicable chronic health conditions and related complications arising from the aging process, which in turn increase the need for multiple treatments. Complexity of the medication regimen is an independent risk factor for missed doses, errors in drug administration, side effects, and drug interactions (Erickson et al., 2017).

The use and overuse of antipsychotic medications in individuals with IDD is another parameter that needs to be closely monitored. Medication regimen reviews for IDD individuals in the community should be conducted on a monthly basis, although there is *not* a law or regulation that requires pharmacist chart review at the community level. It is not uncommon for prescribers or caregivers to utilize sedating medications as "chemical restraints." In long-term-care settings such as nursing homes, consultant pharmacists aggressively patrol for the intentional sedation of nursing home patients with potent antipsychotics without a supporting psychiatric diagnosis. Federal law requires that, on a monthly basis, all patient charts and medication administration records (MARS) are subject to an intensive medication-regimen review (MRR) by a consultant pharmacist. The records are scrutinized for evidence of duplication of therapy, side effects, and adverse drug reactions. Compliance is assessed to make sure all scheduled doses have been administered in a timely manner.

Sometimes there are "hold" parameters that mandate withholding a dose. For example, if the patient is scheduled to receive an antihypertensive medication such as a beta blocker but the blood pressure is already too low, the dose would not be administered. Hypotension (low blood pressure) can lead to heart problems, as well as dizziness and falls. Examples of beta blockers include metoprolol, propranolol, carvedilol, and atenolol. Psychotropic medications are another category of drugs notorious for causing impaired cognition, dizziness, drowsiness, and vertigo, leading to falls in the elderly. In particular, benzodiazepines such as chlordiazepoxide and diazepam significantly increase the risk of cognitive impairment and falls. Falls in long-term-care facilities are considered "sentinel events" and must be reported to the state.

Any observed medication irregularities are immediately flagged by the consultant pharmacist and brought to the attention of the attending physician and the director of nursing. The physician is the boss and always makes the final decision. The pharmacist's recommendations do not have to be implemented if the physician disagrees, but the pharmacist's monthly report does have to be formally acknowledged. If I, as a consultant pharmacist, observe a possible duplication of therapy (the patient is on multiple antidepressants, for example), I never write a rude or sharp recommendation. I write a short, respectful note with my observation that, for example, "this particular patient came back from the hospital and the previous medications were never discontinued. Please evaluate the risk versus benefit for multiple antidepressants." The physician then decides what he or she feels is best.

In the community at large, there are no such legal protections in place to protect vulnerable populations—including IDD individuals and senior citizens—from figuratively and literally falling through the cracks and experiencing the perils of overmedication. One useful publication to which consultant pharmacists frequently refer is the "Beers criteria," named after Dr. Mark Beers. This is essentially a do-not-use list of medications that can precipitate adverse drug events in the elderly. This list is useful not only for long-term-care-facility residents but as a prescribing guide for community living arrangements (CLA), group residential living, and independently living patients. Ultimately, many patients still end up being prescribed some of the Beers criteria drugs, so caregivers must remain vigilant for any potential side effects.

Individuals with IDD live in the community either with their families or, more commonly, under CLA. But it is common for IDD individuals, especially those with dual or multiple diagnoses, to be under the care of multiple prescribers, including PCPs, psychiatrists, and neurologists, each with his or her prescription pad at the ready. Additionally, frequent emergency room visits and subsequent hospital admissions are the norm. Emergency rooms are revolving doors, and it is unlikely that a full medication reconciliation and screening will be conducted by the ER staff, who are already running in circles. Family members and caregivers, including direct-support professionals, should be on high alert to recognize any potential medication-related side effects, such as excessive drowsiness, confusion, and frequent falls, especially since these individuals may not be able to verbally communicate their symptoms.

Once hospitalized, it is unlikely that the patient's PCP will make rounds, but rather the patient will be tended to by various hospitalists on rotating shifts, who will probably never see the patient again after the hospital visit. Upon discharge, yet another set of medications will be prescribed, often with no communication with the individual's PCP and specialists. Meanwhile, drug interactions and side effects are often the underlying reason for the hospital visit in the first place. Hopefully, there will be a proper medication reconciliation, where preadmission medications are compared to in-house medication regimens and to discharge medications. Medication reconciliation provides the individuals, families, and outside doctors and pharmacies with some type of guidance regarding which subset of the old medications to discontinue, which medications to continue, and which new medications need to be started.

Persons with IDD are typically cared for in the primary care setting (where overprescribing is already the norm) and are prescribed twice as many medications as those without IDD (Erickson et al., 2017). There are not enough primary care providers out there to spend adequate time on prevention, and, to repeat, a typical doctor visit lasts less than fifteen minutes. Primary care doctors, like many others, are overworked and stressed out by managed care. Those persons with IDD may not be able to effectively communicate any potential adverse reactions and/or medication side effects to their caregivers and providers. On many occasions, the treatment for one disease state induces another disease state (or symptoms that mimic another disease state) that necessitates even more medications being prescribed. We get caught up in a vicious cycle of polypharmacy and side effects with still more drugs being prescribed to combat the side effects of the previously prescribed drugs—and so on and so on and so on. Having a consultant pharmacist who is not employed by the dispensing pharmacy independently review the charts and medication administration records of all IDD individuals can help reduce medication misadventures.

Direct-support staff must be trained to observe and report any unusual signs and symptoms on behalf of their individuals. Practitioners must assess the risk versus the benefit of each medication before choosing what medications to prescribe. Practitioners should also be willing to *deprescribe* any medications that are producing adverse drug reactions or simply do not have a supporting diagnosis.

In many cases, a gradual dose reduction (GDR), rather than the complete discontinuation of a potentially beneficial medication, might be appropriate. The very same drugs that are therapeutic in lower doses are often toxic in higher doses, especially in vulnerable populations that may have diminished liver and kidney function as the result of advanced age and/or comorbidities. Pharmacies provide an essential health care function by filling prescriptions for sick patients. However, as a consultant pharmacist, I am always vigilant for GDR opportunities to help seniors and persons with IDD avoid medication misadventures.

Independently Living Seniors

Those seniors who reside independently are at the mercy of the less regulated world of retail pharmacy. Retail chain pharmacies make money by using the fastfood model. Pharmacists must fill as many prescriptions as they possibly can in the shortest amount of time with a skeleton crew of workers. The less money spent on pharmacy staffing, the more profit, the higher the stock price, and the happier the shareholders. It is not profitable for chain pharmacies to conduct free nontangible medication regimen reviews for their patients. Consultant pharmacists do not routinely review charts or profiles for those senior citizens who live on their own in homes or apartments. Consequently, independently living seniors are at a very high risk for polypharmacy and suffer greatly from duplications of therapy and adverse drug reactions. Medication misadventures are the cause of many emergency room visits and subsequent hospital admissions. Upon discharge from the hospital, many elderly patients have their discharge prescriptions filled, take them home, dump them into the basket with all their preadmission medications, and take them all together. I have seen this happen numerous times. The patients then go back to the pharmacy when their supplies run low, and they refill *all* their medications. They refill the preadmission medications if they still have refills on the bottle, and they also refill all the new medications. Now we have a little old lady, or perhaps a World War II veteran, with a mixture of as many as twenty prescription bottles. We have the brand name of one drug and the generic of another drug that duplicates the first drug. We have a mixture of old and new medications from multiple doctors and multiple pharmacies. We have polypharmacy.

I can remember, decades ago, being a pharmacy student and filling prescriptions at my father's pharmacy in Philadelphia, then delivering them to senior citizens in various high-rise apartment buildings. Patients would often sit me down at the kitchen table and ask me dozens of questions about the many prescription bottles for everything from blood pressure medications to potent anticoagulants like Coumadin (warfarin). There would often be multiple and duplicate bottles from a multitude of pharmacies, all lined up across the windowsill or in a basket on the table. I would open my reference book (no smartphones back then) and cross-check all the drugs for side effects, interactions, and duplications of therapy. Medication mismanagement is a significant contributor to senior citizens being forced into long-term-care facilities, often resulting in significant loss of independence. Do we really want a World War II veteran who saved the world from tyranny to die from a medication misadventure? I hope not.

The more work that is forced upon the salaried chain pharmacist, the more money that goes toward the bottom line for the shareholders. Any retail druggist will tell you that he or she has a blue-collar job, running about the pharmacy lab juggling prescription bottles, fielding multiple phone calls simultaneously, and even unloading the weekly delivery truck. He or she comes home with aching feet and back, just the same as auto mechanics or contractors do. It's all accomplished for a flat salary with no overtime, no lunch breaks, and full bladders. One of the first concepts taught in pharmacy school is the Patient's Bill of Rights: the *right* drug prescribed at the *right* dose to the *right* patient and given via the *right* route of administration at the *right* time. Patients are often denied these rights. Errors are made, and patients die as a consequence of these errors.

As a pharmacist I have seen many near misses, and I personally and professionally advise the reader to fight for his or her "rights." Always know what medications have been prescribed for you and your loved ones. The prescriber must properly issue a legible handwritten prescription or properly select the correct menu choices to populate an electronic prescription. E-scripts eliminate the risk of illegible handwriting, which has plagued the health care system since the dawn of time. But prescribing errors are still possible since prescribers must use drop-down menus to select drugs and dosages. It is easy to inadvertently tap the wrong menu choice with the stylus, especially when managed care is making everyone work faster and jump through hoops all day long. The pharmacy and pharmacist are responsible for properly processing the e-scripts for the correct patients and dispensing the correct product with the correct instructions. Never assume your prescription has been written or filled correctly. Google it before you fill it, and google it after you fill it. You must know what your medication is being prescribed for, and you must know what your medication should look like.

Every patient is entitled to receive the right drug, prescribed for the right diagnosis, dispensed in the right dose, administered at the right time, given via the right route of administration.

You can look up the pill image and compare it to what you have. If the pills do not appear to be the same, investigate further to make sure that there has not been a prescribing error or a dispensing error. You should also download a free application called Epocrates for your smartphone that allows you to input the color of a tablet or capsule, a description of its shape and size, and the markings on the front and back. Plug in the data, and the app tells you the name and strength of the medication in your bottle. Now you can double-check your own prescriptions in case the overworked mail-order pharmacist was not provided sufficient time by the greedy PBM. Also make a photocopy or take a cell phone picture of your prescription before mailing it or submitting it to the pharmacy. Even if your health care team does everything perfectly, your nonbioequivalent generic prescription drug was probably manufactured in China or India and may just kill you anyway.

Gone are the days when pharmacists had to type one label at time manually on an old-fashioned typewriter. Today, high-tech laser printers spit out hundreds of prescription drug labels an hour. The tiny print on pharmacy labels is difficult for anyone to read, especially the elderly. Like all our other faculties, our vision gets progressively worse as we age. The Veterans Administration has taken steps to address this issue by introducing easier-to-read prescription drug labels. With the demographics of an aging population, it only makes sense that we should make our prescription drug labels easy for everyone to read and understand. Health literacy varies among populations and individuals, so some patients may not be able to properly interpret and understand the information on the label. There may also be cultural or language barriers that interfere with proper medication usage. For example, California law mandates that pharmacies offer translation services in Spanish, Chinese, Vietnamese, Korean, and Russian. Pharmacy labels are the last safety net between medication errors and adverse drug effects, and it's important that all, and especially senior citizens, are properly educated on how to safely take their medications.

PRIMARY PREVENTION

Primary prevention focuses on reducing the development of sickness and disease. Smoking-prevention and smoking-cessation programs, for example, can help reduce the occurrence of many diseases, including cancer, emphysema, and chronic bronchitis. Primary prevention emphasizes education and can prevent the disease or condition before it sets in by focusing on behaviors such as getting all recommended immunizations, adopting a healthy lifestyle including diet and exercise, and undertaking other proactive measures. The diabetes epidemic is a great example of how lifestyle modifications can reduce risk. Type 2 diabetes is a predictable, progressive disease with strong genetic links. While *both* types of diabetes cause the long-term complications of blindness, kidney disease, and amputations, as well as circulatory and cardiovascular problems, type 2 diabetes is preceded by a prediabetes phase. The complications of diabetes often set in during the prediabetes phase, long before individuals are aware that they have diabetes and often many years before an actual diagnosis of type 2 diabetes is made (ADA, 2019). For this reason, regular screenings, particularly for those who are high-risk, represent potentially lifesaving interventions and are an important component of prevention in public health.

Health Promotion

Primary prevention can often be achieved through health education. In the case of type 2 diabetes, for example, there are nonmodifiable risk factors, such as family history, advanced age, and ethnicity, that we have no control over. Sedentary lifestyles and obesity are the main modifiable risk factors that drive the type 2 diabetes epidemic. The social determinants of health care play significant roles here as well. For example, some people reside in food deserts and lack basic access to full-service supermarkets with fresh fruits, vegetables, fish, and poultry. Others simply do not have adequate knowledge of basic nutrition principles. By targeting healthy individuals who are not yet sick as well as members of high-risk groups, public health professionals can work toward prevention.

Education about healthy diet and regular exercise are key factors in the primary prevention of type 2 diabetes. The National Health and Nutrition Examination Survey (NHANES) is primary prevention and represents a policy designed to assess the health and nutritional status of adults and children in the United States. The mandatory coverage for immunizations by the ACA is another example of primary prevention.

Secondary Prevention

Secondary prevention focuses on screening and early detection. Early detection of most diseases permits rapid intervention and improves health outcomes while decreasing morbidity and mortality. Colonoscopies, mammograms, cholesterol screenings, blood pressure monitoring, and blood sugar screenings are some examples of secondary prevention. The medicalization of the term *prediabetes* is an example of policy that transformed the jargon of "borderline diabetes" or "a touch of the sugar" into an officially recognized and billable disease.

There now exist specific numerical values for both fasting blood glucose as well as hemoglobin A1C that corresponds to a diagnosis of prediabetes. A diagnosis of prediabetes sends an ominous message to the patient that the time has arrived for lifestyle modification. Additionally, it allows primary care providers to get paid and to refer patients to other providers (dietitians, exercise specialists, etc.) for interventions. Other examples of secondary prevention include mammograms and colonoscopies. ACA is an example of a policy that promotes secondary prevention by mandating that certain screenings are covered with zero co-pays. Those patients with prediabetes who fail to reverse their disease via secondary prevention are destined to progress to a diagnosis of type 2 diabetes. The administration of insulin prevents or delays the progression of morbidity and mortality associated with diabetes.

Tertiary Prevention

Despite our best efforts, some people will still be diagnosed with diseases. In the manifestation of diabetes, we can still prevent or delay the complications associated with the disease by administering oral medications and/or insulin and conducting blood-glucose monitoring. Diabetes is the leading cause of blindness, end-stage renal disease, and lower-extremity amputations. As such, tertiary prevention is of the utmost importance in avoiding these pitfalls. We can visit our physicians on a regular basis for checkups, treatments, and prescription renewals. Hypertension (high blood pressure) is a commonly occurring comorbidity associated with diabetes. We can advise those with hypertension to follow a sodium-restricted diet and administer antihypertensive medications to them. In addition to medications, other clinical measures may also be necessary, such as monitoring blood pressure with a sphygmomanometer. Diabetes is the seventh-leading cause of death in the United States. Additionally, it contributes to heart disease, the number one cause of death (CDC, 2020). In order to minimize the morbidity and mortality inflicted by diabetes, patients need to be reminded to see their primary care providers and specialists on a regular basis for routine monitoring of their blood glucose and their A1C. Many patients with diabetes often check their own blood glucose at home on a routine basis.

THE DIABETES PANDEMIC

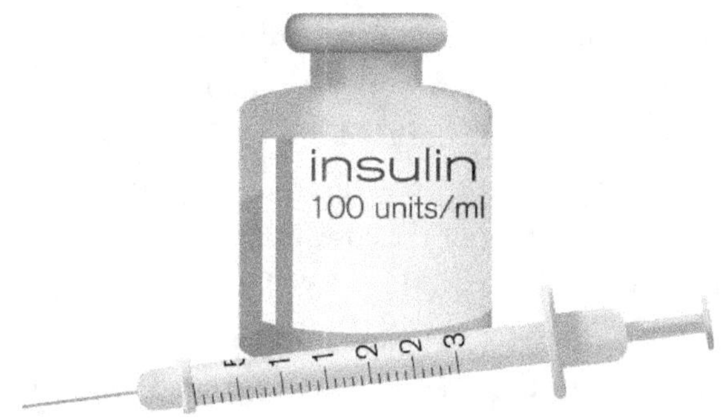

Diabetes is a chronic, debilitating disease that occurs when the pancreas becomes incapable of producing adequate amounts of the hormone insulin and/or when the body cannot effectively take up and utilize the insulin that is produced. Diabetes is classified as either type 1 or type 2, depending on the above criteria.

Diabetes is an epidemic afflicting over thirty million people in the United States and a pandemic with upward of five hundred million people affected worldwide (ADA, 2020; WHO, 2018). The prevalence of diabetes domestically and globally is approaching 10 percent, with one in every twelve people on the planet affected (International Diabetes Federation, 2017). According to the CDC, medical costs for people with diabetes are typically more than twice as high as for people without diabetes. Patients with diabetes spend thousands of extra dollars on medication and pharmacy expenses compared to those without diabetes. It has been estimated that close to $600 billion is spent annually on diabetes in the United States. This represents one out of every nine US economy dollars. Diabetes is frequently reported as the seventh-leading cause of death in the United States, but this statistic likely reflects underreporting.

With such an overwhelming global prevalence of diabetes, it is imperative that the reader have a basic understanding and appreciation of how insulin works in the human body. Additionally, many readers may not realize that the discovery and isolation of insulin, as well as the availability of the commercially prepared product, is a relatively recent event that should not be taken for granted (Davidson, 1981).

Insulin is a hormone that facilitates the entry of glucose from the bloodstream into the cells, where it is needed for energy. The best analogy to demonstrate this concept is envisioning insulin as the key that unlocks the cells so that glucose can enter the cells (Bliss, 1982). Insulin works in conjunction with other hormones, including glucagon, to maintain consistent blood-glucose levels.

Type 1 diabetes strikes quickly and unpredictably and is characterized by a swift and complete destruction of the insulin-producing pancreatic beta cells. The scientific community believes that type 1 diabetes results from a genetic predisposition plus an exposure to an environmental factor. In a person who is genetically predisposed to the disease, environmental triggers are thought to cause an autoimmune response that leads to destruction of the pancreatic beta cells. Despite the swift clinical presentation of type 1 diabetes, there is typically a long period of time prior to diagnosis during which immune markers are present and beta cell destruction is occurring.

Prior to 1921, a diagnosis of type 1 diabetes was a sentence to a slow death by starvation. Imagine an automobile with an empty fuel tank parked at the gas pump. If the gasoline is not pumped into the automobile's gas tank, the car is starved for fuel, and the vehicle goes nowhere. The same analogy can be applied to the insulin-glucose relationship. Without insulin on board to facilitate the entry of glucose into the cell, there's too much sugar in the blood. Meanwhile, the patient is deprived of life-sustaining carbohydrates and will die from starvation (Bliss, 1982).

With the insulin-secreting beta cells destroyed, the blood glucose quickly rises to astronomical levels. A patient with type 1 diabetes commonly presents to the emergency room in a state of profound hyperglycemia. Hyperglycemia is the medical term for high blood sugar. When the blood-glucose levels reach around 180 mg/dl, the glucose spills into the urine, creating a condition known as osmotic diuresis. The diuretic effect of the glucose causes frequent urination (polydipsia) and results in severe dehydration and electrolyte depletion. Consequently, the patient becomes very thirsty and begins drinking large quantities of water. The patient also is extremely hungry (polyphagia) because the absence of insulin prevents the utilization of glucose despite extreme hyperglycemia. As a last, desperate measure, the body begins to break down fat as an alternative energy source. This leads to the buildup of ketones in the blood and urine and a condition known as diabetic ketoacidosis.

Doctors had known for years that excessive sugar intake worsened the condition of diabetic patients. Patients were put on very strict diets where sugar intake was kept to a minimum. The strictest of these diets permitted only one thousand calories per day. In fact, patients often starved to death from the diets themselves. Ironically, this type of death was sometimes preferable to the miserable death that diabetes brought (Bliss, 1982).

As early as 1869, a German medical student named Paul Langerhans discovered unique clusters of pancreatic cells with some special yet unknown functions. Eventually they would be identified as the insulin-producing beta cells. This discovery was of such clinical significance that the insulin-producing region of the pancreas was formally named the Islets of Langerhans (Bliss, 1982).

By 1889, scientists knew that the pancreas had at minimum two functions. First, they knew that it produced digestive juices. They also were now certain that the pancreas produced a substance that regulated glucose in the bloodstream. In the summer of 1921, Dr. Frederick Banting and his assistant, Charles Best, worked feverishly in the laboratory at the University of Toronto to isolate the substance that we now know as insulin (Bliss, 1982).

Step one of the research involved the surgical removal of a dog's pancreas. The two men determined that when the pancreas of a dog was removed, the dog's blood sugar rose. The dog developed the classic symptoms of diabetes, including those of polydipsia (thirst), polyphagia (hunger), and polyuria (frequent urination). The dog lost weight and became weaker and weaker. The dog had developed diabetes as a direct result of the pancreatectomy (Bliss, 1982).

Step two involved separating and purifying the pancreatic mixture. This isolate, now called *isletin*, was subsequently injected into the newly diabetic dogs. Amazingly, the dog's blood-glucose levels dropped, and its diabetic symptoms improved. In order to expedite the global availability of insulin, Dr. Banting made the patent available for free. In 1923 Dr. Banting and his team of researchers received the Nobel Prize in Physiology or Medicine for their work. November 14 is Dr. Banting's birthday and is now known as World Diabetes Day.

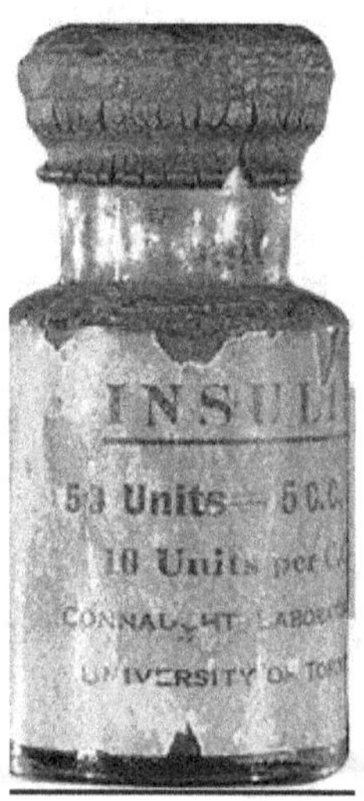

As an animal lover, the author is pained to know that many innocent dogs gave their lives in the quest for isolating what we now call insulin. Even so, countless millions of humans (and pets) have been saved as a result of the experiments. Thanks to the diligence of Banting and Best, individuals with type 1 diabetes are no longer destined to a slow death by starvation. Typically, a frightened and confused patient presents to the emergency room and is admitted to the hospital in a state of severe hyperglycemia, dehydration, electrolyte imbalance, and ketoacidosis. Intravenous insulin and fluids are administered until the patient is rehydrated and the glucose returns to normal levels. Upon discharge, the newly diagnosed type 1 diabetes patient requires a lifetime of exogenous injections (via needle, pen, or pump) for day-to-day survival. Today patients can get on waiting lists for new hearts, livers, and kidneys. Unfortunately, although Banting and Best were thankfully able to isolate insulin, the successful pancreas transplant has yet to become mainstream (Davidson, 1981).

Compared to type 1 diabetes, type 2 diabetes is strongly linked to a variety of risk factors and is more predictable and possibly avoidable. Type 2 diabetes attacks sneakily and silently, and many people are not even aware of the impending doom. Insulin resistance, followed by a progressive beta cell dysfunction, leads to hyperglycemia and a diagnosis of type 2 diabetes. Unfortunately, beta cell failure begins years before the actual type 2 diabetes diagnosis, and the complications begin brewing early on. On the bright side, preventative measures such as regular screenings of fasting blood glucose and hemoglobin A1C can detect a medical condition known as prediabetes early on.

As I have previously mentioned, the relatively new term *prediabetes* is a medicalized version of what used to commonly be referred to as "borderline" diabetic or having "a touch of the sugar," neither of which is acceptable medical terminology and neither of which is billable by medical providers (Conrad, 2007). Prediabetes was assigned its own ICD-10 code, which allows prescribers to initiate treatments that are recognized and billable to insurance providers.

Fortunately, the ACA mandates coverage for such preventive services. When a clinical service such as diabetes screening is covered by insurance, patients are more likely to utilize it, especially when there is no co-pay for the service. Heart disease and obesity are comorbid conditions that frequently accompany diabetes in a vicious cycle, with each condition contributing to the complications of the other. More than one in three Americans and nearly one in five children in our country is obese. The ACA awards millions of dollars to state health departments for the funding of CDC programs targeting diabetes, heart disease and stroke, nutrition, physical activity, obesity, and school health that work in a coordinated fashion to prevent chronic disease by addressing common risk factors. The National Diabetes Prevention Program (NDPP), for example, is a CDC-funded resource to help prevent type 2 diabetes.

https://www.cdc.gov/diabetes/prevention/index.html

The ACA mandates health coverage for everyone, but this does not mean that most Americans can afford the coverage. Even *with* health insurance, the out-of-pocket expenses (premiums, deductibles, and co-pays) for individuals and families with private insurance are often unaffordable. As such, even insured people often have to make the choice between paying for medical expenses and feeding their children. For example, in Coffeyville, Kansas, medical debt collectors decide who gets arrested for not paying up. Citizens, including pregnant women and diabetics, are routinely summoned, sued, and hauled into court by the local hospital, physicians, and ambulance companies. In another example, a pregnant mother in Leroy, Kansas, was arrested because she missed hearings regarding a $230 medical bill. A cancer patient in Indiana was "hauled away in her pajamas" as her family watched helplessly. A man from Utah committed suicide rather than stay in jail over an unpaid ambulance bill. When it comes to the cash, the lawyers (bounty hunters) get a cut of the take. This article is really worth reading; below is a link to the full reference:

https://features.propublica.org/medical-debt/
when-medical-debt-collectors-decide-who-gets-arrested-coffeyville-kansas/

The ACA's emphasis on prevention and public health, over the long haul, could help to alleviate some of these out-of-pocket expenses by decreasing the incidence and prevalence of preventable diseases. Of particular importance are the free screenings and preventive measures such as immunizations that are mandated to be included without any expense to the patient. Of course, the providers are still paid for their services, but patients perceive them as free and are therefore more likely to take advantage of the benefits.

The ACA took one major step forward by establishing the Prevention and Public Health Fund. Repealing the ACA would be like taking two steps back. In a nation such as ours that focuses too much on treatment and not enough on prevention, we cannot afford to lose the only dedicated funding source for prevention and public health, which, by statute, is intended to provide for expanded and sustained national investment in prevention and public health programs to improve health and help restrain the rate of growth in private and public sector health care costs.

Outside the scientific community, few people realize the magnitude and repercussions of diabetes and the complications it causes. When we think of a pandemic, we may envision gruesome scenes such as those of the bubonic plague of the Middle Ages or the contemporary coronavirus that is taking a huge toll globally. But since diabetes is a silent disease, complications such as blindness, kidney disease, and amputations may seemingly appear out of nowhere and can be devastating. Thanks to the rise of medicalization, complications (e.g., diabetic retinopathy, diabetic nephropathy, and diabetic neuropathy) are now recognized with ICD-9 and CPT codes and are covered by insurance for prevention and treatment (Conrad, 2007).

Half a billion people globally are affected by diabetes, correlating with a prevalence of diabetes approaching 10 percent among adults as of 2019. The WHO predicts that diabetes will be the seventh-leading cause of death by 2030, with almost half of all deaths occurring before the age of seventy. Worldwide, the incidence and prevalence of diabetes is rising most rapidly among those in middle- and low-income countries (WHO, 2019). The high glucose concentration is toxic to the blood vessels and nerves, often resulting in long-term complications such as blindness, kidney disease, and nerve damage.

It bears repeating that diabetes is a progressive disease with strong genetic links that causes the long-term complications of blindness, kidney disease, and amputations, as well as circulatory and cardiovascular problems. The complications of diabetes often set in long before an individual is aware that he or she has diabetes. This time period is called prediabetes and may exist for many years before an actual diagnosis is made (ADA, 2019).

There are many risks for developing type 2 diabetes, but the strongest predictor across all populations is obesity. Domestically, there is a higher risk of type 2 diabetes in Latinos, African Americans, and Native Americans (ADA, 2019). These groups also make up a disproportionate share of the poor and uninsured.

Primary Prevention in Diabetes

One of the most applicable examples of primary prevention refers to individuals in a state of prediabetes who are not yet aware because they did not get preventative hemoglobin A1C screenings due to the perceived excessive out-of-pocket expense.

Research has proven unequivocally that prediabetic individuals are already at risk of the complications that accompany a diagnosis of diabetes, even though they have not even been made aware of their diagnosis yet. Again, the preventive care benefits of the ACA can come to the rescue with mandatory covered benefits for a long list of preventive measures, such as hemoglobin A1C screenings that are free to the patient, meaning that there are no co-pays or other out-of-pocket expenses. The provider, of course, still gets paid by the insurance company.

Not filling a prescription for a drug because it is too expensive is a very common scenario that plays out over and over again on a daily basis in almost every pharmacy across America. For example, Mr. Smith, a diabetic individual, makes the choice that he will not fill his prescription for the antibiotic medication to treat a superficial skin infection on the ball of his foot because it doesn't hurt and will ultimately resolve on its own. "It's just not worth the twenty-five-dollar co-pay," he tells the pharmacist as he leaves without filling the prescription. Wrong choice. The simplest, most uncomplicated skin infection, if left untreated in a patient who has diabetes, may quickly progress to a much more serious situation, resulting in a bone infection called osteomyelitis, ultimately leading to hospitalization and requiring intravenous antibiotics. Diabetes, by the nature of the disease, compromises the cardiovascular and circulatory systems, making it likely that the antibiotic will have trouble reaching the site of the infection. Gangrene can set in, leading to partial or total amputation of the toes and/or foot or even more of the extremity.

This scenario plays out all day long in every hospital in every city of every state. The tragic truth regarding Mr. Smith is that, if not for the "gag clauses" mandated by PBMs, the pharmacist may have been able to offer Mr. Smith the same medication for the cash price of ten dollars rather than the insurance price of twenty-five dollars. Mr. Smith would have filled the prescription and cured the infection while it was still in its superficial and curable stage. Thanks to recently passed legislation authored by Representative Earl L. "Buddy" Carter (R-GA), gag clauses may now become a thing of the past. Cheers to this hero.

https://buddycarter.house.gov/news/documentsingle.aspx?DocumentID=3529

THE OPIOID EPIDEMIC

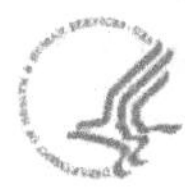

Office of the Secretary

Washington DC 20201

DETERMINATION THAT A PUBLIC HEALTH EMERGENCY EXISTS

As a result of the consequences of the opioid crisis affecting our Nation, on this date and after consultation with public health officials as necessary, I, Eric D. Hargan, Acting Secretary of Health and Human Services, pursuant to the authority vested in me under section 319 of the Public Health Service Act, do hereby determine that a public health emergency exists nationwide.

10/26/2017
Date

/s/
Eric D. Hargan
Acting Secretary

The Spanish flu of 1918 wiped out upward of 100 million people. Scientific advances such as immunizations, clean water and sanitation, and the discovery of antibiotics had (up until the current COVID-19 pandemic) put a stop to contagious plagues and pandemics, allowing us to live longer. Hopefully, we will have a COVID-19 immunization available in the near future. As this book goes to print, over 328,000 persons have died from COVID-19 worldwide. Even though COVID-19 has overtaken the headlines in the media, the opioid epidemic (while not infectious) rages on. According to the CDC, over 130 people die from opioid overdoses in the United States every day. Examples of opioids include the illegal drug heroin, synthetic opioids such as fentanyl, and pain relievers available legally by prescription such as oxycodone, hydrocodone, codeine, morphine, and others.

All opioids are chemically related and interact with opioid receptors on nerve cells in the body and brain. When the body is in pain, neurotransmitters such as endorphins attach to the opioid receptors in the brain and elsewhere. Opioid drugs mimic that reaction. With too much of an opioid drug, the body overdoses. Opioid pain relievers produce euphoria in addition to pain relief and can therefore be abused when taken more frequently or in a higher quantity than prescribed. Even when prescribed by a doctor, opioid usage frequently leads to dependence, addiction, overdose, and death. When someone overdoses, naloxone can be given by injection or squirted into someone's nose to rapidly reverse opioid overdose. Narcan (naloxone) nasal spray is easily administered by relatives, caregivers, or passersby. It can very quickly restore normal respiration to a person whose breathing has slowed or stopped as a result of overdosing with heroin or prescription opioid pain medications. Naloxone is an opioid antagonist that works by binding to opioid receptors, thus reversing and blocking the effects of other opioids. Naloxone is extremely effective and can start working in minutes, depending on the dosage and potency of the drug taken. For more powerful opioids such as fentanyl, it may take several doses. Naloxone is not addictive and has few side effects. The drug works on someone only if there are opioids in his or her system already. It cannot prevent an overdose and cannot work on any other type of drug overdose. However, the effects of naloxone wear off quickly, and the victim may lapse back into respiratory depression because the opiate is still in his or her system. Therefore, it is crucial to also call 911 or get the patient to the emergency room immediately after administering Narcan.

https://www.drugabuse.gov/related-topics/opioid-overdose-reversal-naloxone-narcan-evzio

Counterfeit narcotic drug products from across the globe flood the US marketplace and are becoming increasingly deadly. One of the reasons that the opioid epidemic has become so deadly is that many medications sold online and on the street are laced with toxic contaminants, including counterfeit and synthetic fentanyl, carfentanil, chalk dust, and antifreeze. It is tragic enough that legitimate opioids are killing us, but these highly potent additives kill instantly, and they can even be unintentionally absorbed through the skin. The victims of the opioid epidemic are not intentionally killing themselves. They naively think they are simply getting their next high, having no clue that they may be dead in a few seconds. Even law enforcement officers have succumbed to these deadly toxins via external contact and have needed Narcan (naloxone) revival.

It is vital that all communities expand the availability of Narcan to all patients, caregivers, and family members and train them to save a life. Wider availability of Narcan can help reverse the trend of decreasing life expectancy in the United States. The opioid crisis has been overshadowed by the current COVID-19 situation, but the president has previously acknowledged the public health emergency created by the staggering number of opioid-related deaths. The Department of Health and Human Services (HHS) unveiled a five-point opioid strategy with the five following priorities:

- Improve access to prevention, treatment, and recovery support services

- Target the availability and distribution of overdose-reversing drugs such as Narcan

- Strengthen public health data reporting and collection

- Support cutting-edge research on addiction and pain

- Advance the practice of pain management

THE OPIOID EPIDEMIC BY THE NUMBERS

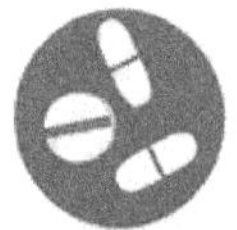

130+
People died every day from
opioid-related drug overdoses[3]
(estimated)

10.3 m
People misused
prescription opioids in 2018[1]

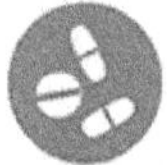

47,600
People died from
overdosing on opioids[2]

2.0 million
People had an opioid use
disorder in 2018[1]

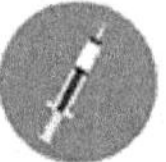

808,000
People used heroin
in 2018[1]

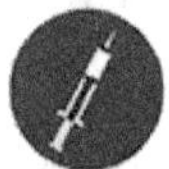

81,000
People used heroin
for the first time[1]

2 million
People misused
prescription opioids
for the first time[1]

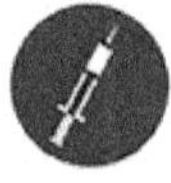

15,349
Deaths attributed to
overdosing on heroin
(in 12-month period
ending February 2019)[2]

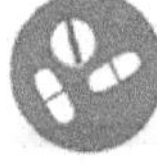

32,656
Deaths attributed to overdosing
on synthetic opioids other than
methadone (in 12-month period
ending February 2019)[2]

SOURCES

1. 2019 National Survey on Drug Use and Health. Mortality in the United States, 2018
2. NCHS Data Brief No. 329, November 2018
3. NCHS, National Vital Statistics System. Estimates for 2018 and 2019 are based on
provisional data.

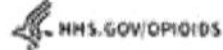

THE PATENT MEDICINE ERA: 1860–1920

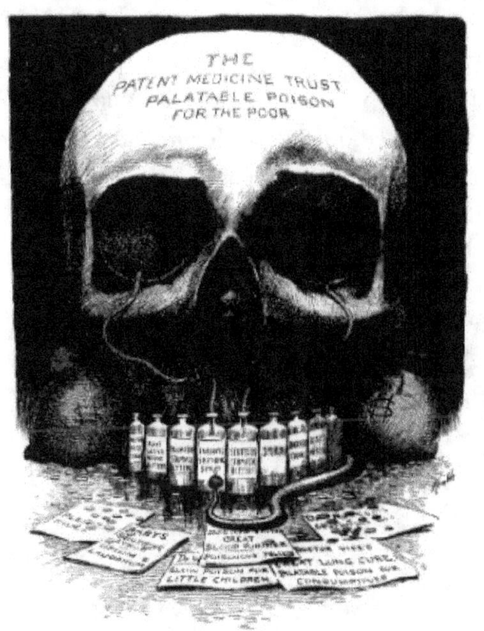

In 1820 the United States Pharmacopeia (USP) became the first official compendium of the United States. Doctors and pharmacists could refer to the USP for information and guidelines regarding strength and purity of various pharmaceutical products. The nineteenth century brought an eruption in patent medications and quack remedies. Any salve, syrup, potion, pill, or tonic could be sold on the open market without a doctor's prescription, and any therapeutic claim could be made, no matter how outrageous. These useless products often contained harmful ingredients that were usually unknown to patients and physicians. There were no oversights or regulations regarding accurate and honest labeling. These patent medications were frequently counterfeited or adulterated with unproven, diluted, or inactive ingredients. There was no FDA to protect the public, so these toxic products were often hawked directly to the unwary public by traveling street salesmen or "medicine men" (who knew nothing about medicine) rather than ordered by physicians. The medicine man had the job of persuading sick people to buy his particular brand of snake oil from among the hundreds available in the marketplace.

Americans during this period were not very knowledgeable about medicine and science. Patients wanted quick fixes for medical problems that they did not necessarily comprehend. Doctors were scarce and were not always knowledgeable or trustworthy. Hospitals were traditionally considered scary places where people went to die.

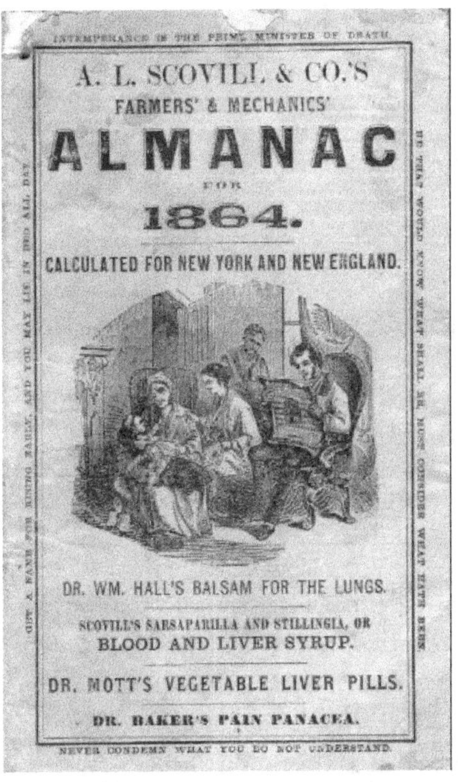

Patent medicines were often marketed in almanacs as cure-alls to provide quick, convenient, and cheap relief from arthritis, depression, mental illness, women's problems, men's problems, indigestion, liver problems, and lack of hair growth. Almanacs, free publications that contained weather forecasts, horoscopes, and health advice, provided the perfect vehicle to get the attention of a captive audience desperate to find remedies for their ailments. Feeling better was not necessarily the result of the patent medicine's therapeutic properties but rather related to the fact that many patent medicines were laden with addictive drugs such as opium, morphine, cocaine, and alcohol. The phrase "patent medicine" comes from the late seventeenth-century marketing of medicinal elixirs. Few, if any, of the concoctions were actually patented. Patenting one of these quack remedies would have required public disclosure of its ingredients, which most promoters wished to avoid because they often caused more harm than good.

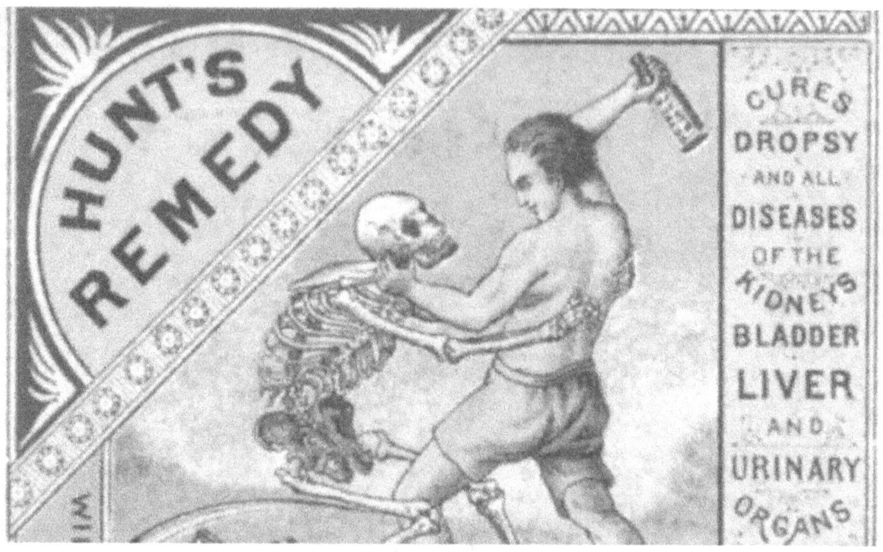

Advertising campaigns in publications such as *Good Housekeeping*, *Ladies' Home Journal*, and *Collier's* kept these patent medications in the public view and instilled the belief that no disease was beyond cure. The manufacturers of such remedies created trademarks and product branding to distinguish their highly profitable products from the crowd of competitors. Thanks to aggressive marketing and the absence of drug regulation, the patent medicine trade was making manufacturers and traveling salesmen rich. Many people relied on patent medicines out of fear and distrust of the contemporary medical establishment.

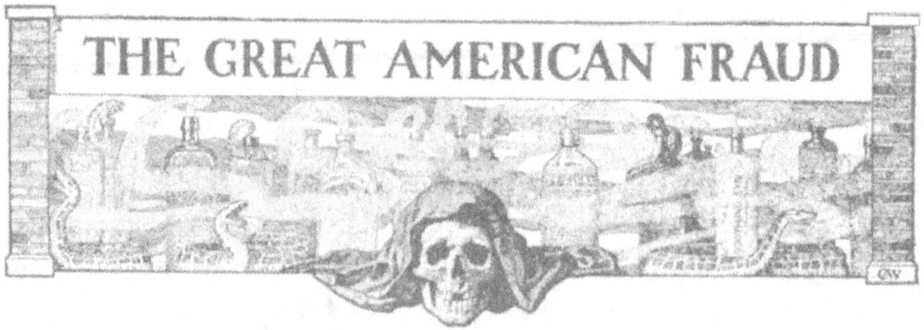

Samuel Hopkins Adams was a muckraker who began his career as a reporter for the *New York Sun*, where he worked from 1891 to 1900. Later, he worked as a freelance writer for *McClure's* magazine. Adams soon gained a reputation for publishing articles exposing public health injustices in the United States. In 1905 *Collier's* contracted with Adams to write articles on the patent drug industry. In his series of articles entitled "The Great American Fraud," Adams exposed many of the false claims made about patent medicines, pointing out that in many scenarios these nostrums were damaging the health of the people using them. Like Sinclair, Adams's investigative work was instrumental in the passage of the Pure Food and Drug Act of 1906. This milestone marked the beginning of federal drug regulation. In 1911, the Supreme Court ruled that the prohibition of falsifications referred only to the ingredients of the patent medicines. This permitted manufacturers to continue to promote greatly embellished claims about the curative powers of their mysterious potions. Adams then went on in 1914 to write *The Clarion*, which exposed unscrupulous newspaper advertising practices and prompted a series of consumer-protection articles in the *New York Tribune*. Adams (1905) wrote, "If there is no limit to the gullibility of the public on one hand, there is apparently none to the cupidity of the newspapers on the other."

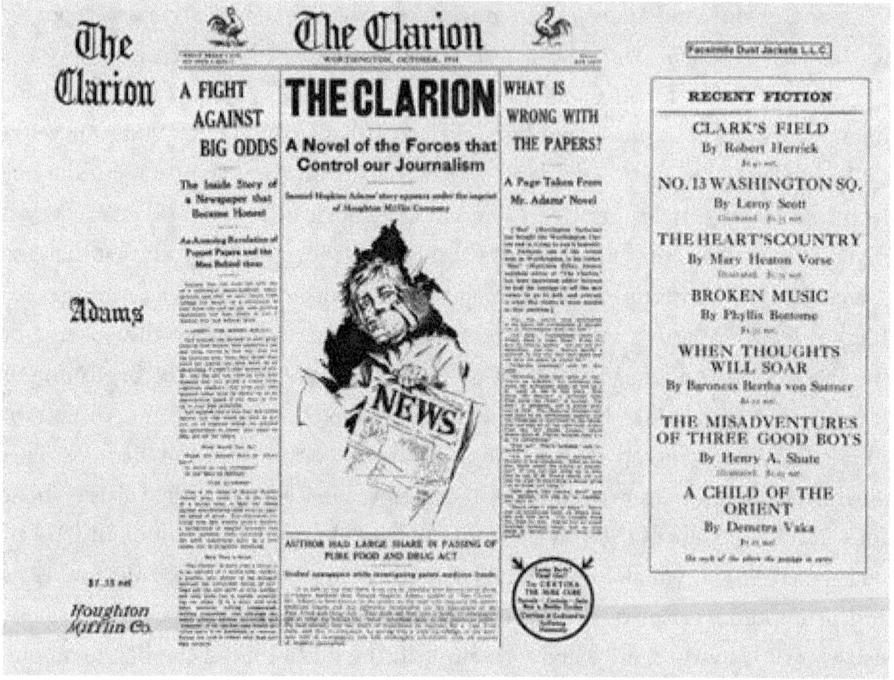

Many panaceas from the patent medicine era live on today in brands such as Luden's Cough Drops, Smith Brothers Cough Drops, Lydia E. Pinkham's Vegetable Compound, Fletcher's Castoria, Phillips' Milk of Magnesia, Vicks VapoRub, Doan's Pills, Bromo-Seltzer, and others. Though sold at high prices, many of these products were made from cheap ingredients. Their composition was well known within the pharmacy world, and pharmacists manufactured and sold (for a slightly lower price) medicines of almost identical composition.

Competition was fierce, so to protect profits, the quack-medicine advertisements emphasized brand names and urged the public to "accept no substitutes." The advertisements of the day speak to the creative appeals that were hawked to the general public. Some of today's over-the-counter products were once marketed as patent medicines but have been reformulated and are no longer making medicinal claims. In many of the recipes, the original ingredients have been changed to remove drugs.

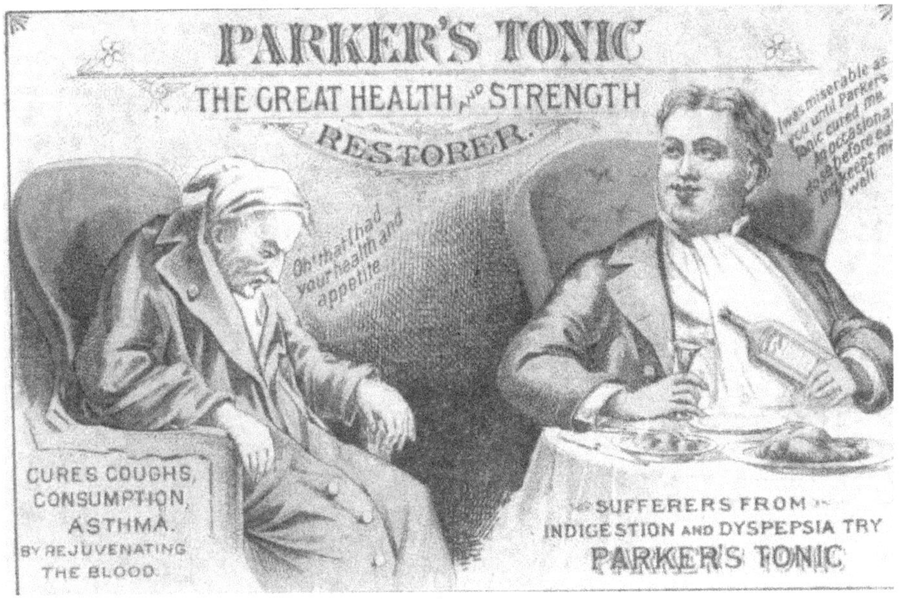
PARKER'S TONIC
THE GREAT HEALTH AND STRENGTH
RESTORER.
Oh that I had your health and appetite
I was miserable as you until Parkers Tonic cured me. I occasionally take it before eating and it keeps me well
CURES COUGHS, CONSUMPTION, ASTHMA. BY REJUVENATING THE BLOOD.
SUFFERERS FROM INDIGESTION AND DYSPEPSIA TRY PARKER'S TONIC

THE CIVIL WAR ERA

SNAKE-OIL LINIMENT
RELIEVES INSTANTANEOUSLY
AND CURES HEADACHE, NEURALGIA, TOOTHACHE, EARACHE, BACKACHE, SWELLINGS, SPRAINS, SORE CHEST, SWELLING of the THROAT, CONTRACTED CORDS and MUSCLES, STIFF JOINTS, WRENCHES, DISLOCATIONS, CUTS and BRUISES.

It Quickly takes out the Soreness and Inflammation from Corns, Bunions, Insect and Reptile Bites.

The best External Preparation for BYCICLISTS and ATHLETES. It makes the Muscles supple and Relaxes the Cords. Loosens the Joints and gives a feeling of Freshness and Vigor to the whole System.

SNAKE-OIL LINIMENT CURES ALL ACHES AND PAINS.

If you are suffering from Rheumatism, ALWAYS take LA-CAS-KA internally for the Blood and so SNAKE-OIL LINIMENT externally. When used together we GUARANTEE A CURE in every instance or MONEY REFUNDED.

If You Are Afflicted With DEAFNESS
Get Our Specially Prepared
PURE Rattlesnake Oil

With the Civil War raging, people were hungry for information concerning the battles and were voraciously reading all of the newspapers and magazines they could get their hands on. The purveyors of patent medicines used this to their advantage and advertised in all the periodicals of the era. Most of the soldiers that died during the Civil War perished due to disease, not from battle. The makers of these patent medicines also preyed upon the public's extreme fear of epidemic diseases such as typhoid, typhus, yellow fever, scurvy, malaria, tuberculosis, smallpox, and cholera. The US government got in on the lucrative patent medicine action as well, taxing the nostrums to help fund the Civil War and, later, the Spanish-American War efforts and the repaying of military debts.

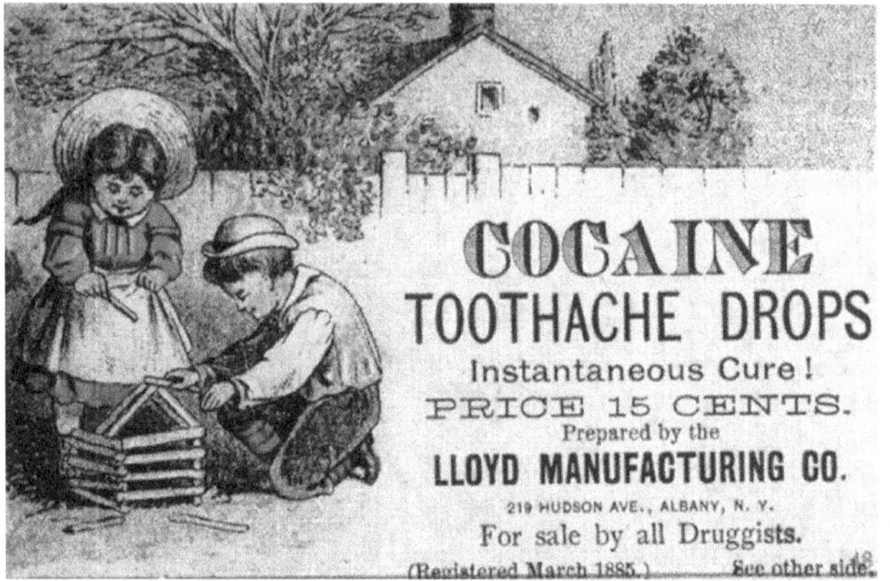

Harvey Wiley

In 1883 Harvey Washington Wiley arrived as chief chemist of the division of chemistry in the Department of Agriculture. Wiley expanded the bureau's food adulteration studies. Wiley became known as the Crusading Chemist and the Father of the Pure Food and Drugs Act. From 1887 to 1902, Wiley published a ten-part study entitled *Foods and Food Adulterants*. He also conducted his now-famous "poison-squad" experiments, in which healthy volunteers ingested samples of unknown or questionable food additives to determine their safety for human consumption.

In late 1901 thirteen children died after being given a tainted diphtheria vaccine in Saint Louis. The Biologics Control Act became law the following year. Strict licensing and labeling requirements were established to ensure the purity and safety of serums, vaccines, and similar products used to prevent and treat diseases in humans. Congress also allocated $5,000 for Wiley's Bureau of Chemistry (formerly the Department of Chemistry) to begin investigations into the health effects of chemical food preservatives and colors on digestion and health. Wiley gathered a group of volunteers who were to eat foods with established concentrations of preservatives and whose physical characteristics were carefully measured and recorded over a specified time period. The media named the group Wiley's "poison squad" and followed the human guinea pigs over the course of their long experiment. The nation was watching as Dr. Wiley's studies exposed the widespread problem of adulteration in the food supply. Citizens began waking up to the realization that the country was in dire need of federal food and drug legislation to protect the public from consuming potentially dangerous substances.

The Wiley Act of 1906

The Pure Food and Drug Act, also known as the Wiley Act, was strongly endorsed by President Theodore Roosevelt and represented the first federal statute targeting misbranding. In addition to mandating federal inspections of meat products, the Wiley Act also marked the beginning of the end for the patent medicine industry. The manufacture, sale, or transportation of adulterated food products and poisonous patent medicines was now forbidden. Questionable products were subject to seizure, and the responsible parties could now be held legally accountable and prosecuted. Still, the Wiley Act exerted authority only *after* drugs were already on the market. This law focused primarily on the accuracy of product labeling as opposed to any type of premarket approvals. Food and drug labels were now mandated not to contain any inaccurate or misleading information. Ingredients now had to be printed on labels, with false claims toned down and advertising more truthful.

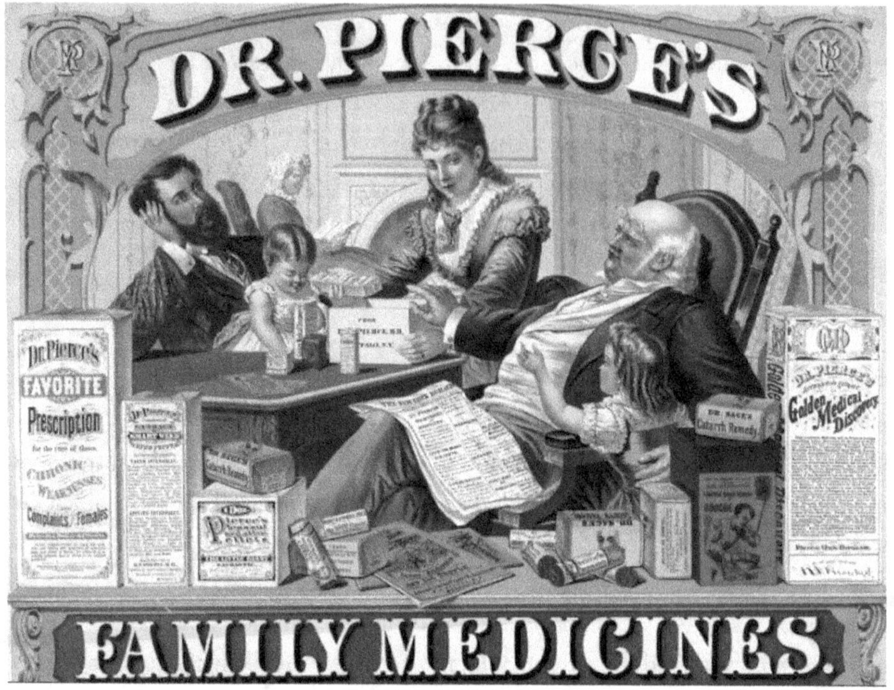

The gold standards of reference at this time were now the United States Pharmacopoeia (USP) and the National Formulary (NF). Any deviations from strength, quality, and purity as specified in the USP and NF had to be listed on product labels. The *disclosure* of eleven dangerous ingredients, including as alcohol, heroin, and cocaine, was also mandated by the Wiley Act. The act still did *not* ban the inclusion of such toxic ingredients; even so, it curbed some of the misleading, overstated, and fraudulent claims that appeared on the labels. The Pure Food and Drug Act would provide the FDA with the necessary authority on certain matters by setting standards, procedures, and criminal and civil enforcement powers.

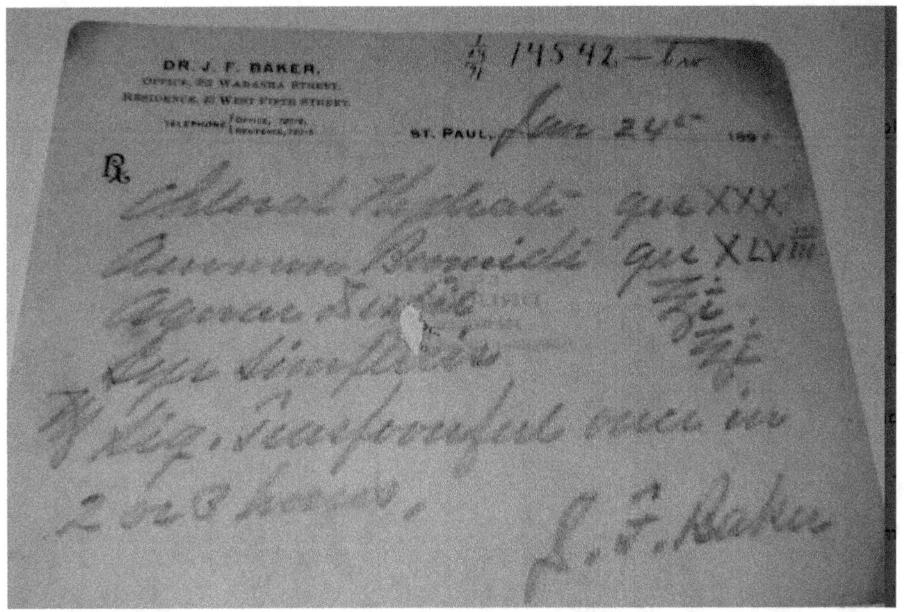

1891 prescription for chloral hydrate

The Wiley Act of 1906 paved the way for the passage of the 1938 Food, Drug, and Cosmetic Act, which still (as amended) governs the manufacturing of today's foods, pharmaceuticals, and cosmetics. The reader must realize that it was the corruption in the US food and agriculture industries that was the driving force behind the Wiley Act.

Therefore, we are obligated to acknowledge FDA's vital role in protecting us from potentially dangerous foods. Food regulation was the precursor to drug regulation, and we all need to remain wary of the foods we consume because even with all our advances in microbiology and food safety, botulism and salmonella outbreaks still occur to this day. People still die from food poisoning, just as they die from medication-related issues, and both topics require our continued vigilance.

The Wiley Act did not require any specific information, such as the name of the food, the ingredients, quantity, or the names and addresses of the manufacturer and distributor. Without the name of the food or knowledge of the ingredients, who would know what he or she was consuming? Even though FDA had already defined over two hundred standards of identity for food even before the Wiley Act was passed, the act did not officially give FDA authority to set food standards.

During the time that Wiley presided over the Bureau of Chemistry, the regulatory emphasis focused on foods. Upon Wiley's resignation in 1912, the agency began to move more toward drug regulation, including patent medicines. During the patent medicine era, many drugs were labeled with false therapeutic claims that were specifically intended to defraud the naive public. The bureau seized many batches of adulterated and misbranded drugs during the 1920s and 1930s. Still, the 1906 law only prohibited misleading claims about ingredients. Many unworthy products still found their way into the marketplace, as there were no restrictions on therapeutic claims (Hutt & Merrill, 2007).

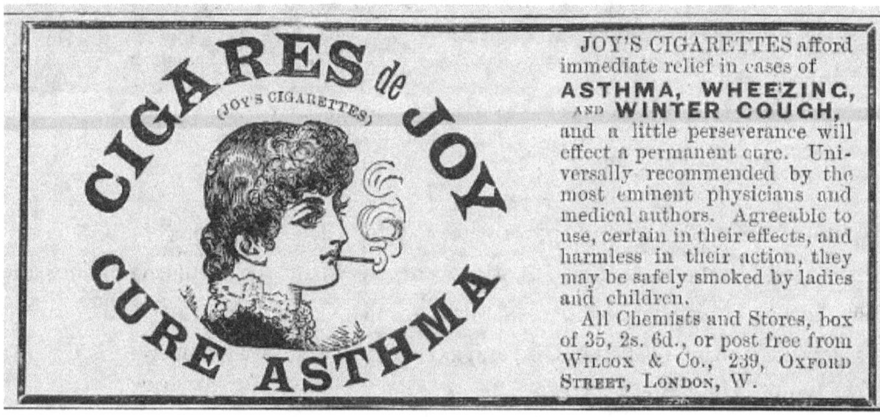

The End of the Patent Medicine Era

In 1937 S. E. Massengill Company introduced a raspberry-flavored liquid antibiotic formulation called Elixir Sulfanilamide. An agent called diethylene glycol, a highly toxic chemical analogue of antifreeze, was used to solubilize the sulfa antibiotic. In short order, over one hundred people, mostly children, died as a result of consuming this product. Tragedy, especially when it causes death or bodily harm to a large number of people, often leads to improvements in the law.

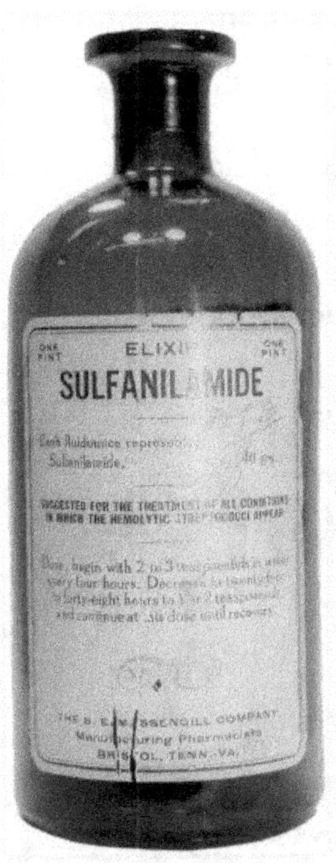

Shortly after this therapeutic disaster, President Franklin Delano Roosevelt signed the Food, Drug, and Cosmetic Act on June 25, 1938. This new law had more teeth and replaced the Pure Food and Drug Act of 1906. Authority now rested with the FDA to oversee the safety of food, drugs, and cosmetics and to *prevent harm before it occurred*. Now, all new drugs had to be tested by their manufacturers for safety. The results of such tests were to be submitted to the government. The drug would then be approved by way of a new drug application (NDA). In summary, not only does a drug have to work; it also has to be safe. It seems quite logical that if the risk of taking a pharmaceutical product exceeds any potential therapeutic benefit, then that particular drug should not be permitted for sale to the public.

A single comprehensive statute—the 1938 Federal Food, Drug, and Cosmetic Act, as amended—provides the basic legal framework controlling the activities of foods, drugs, cosmetics, and medical devices. A tragedy similar to the

Sulfanilamide diethylene glycol disaster was repeated again in 2006 when one hundred people in Panama died after taking cough syrup containing a Chinese-made sweetener tainted with industrial diethylene glycol (Lizcano, 2016).

Fast-forward to the year 2020, and unproven coronavirus cures are running FDA in regulatory circles, with fake doctors taking to the internet peddling unproven nostrums reminiscent of the patent medicine era. According to the *Wall Street Journal*, "The Federal Trade Commission and the Food and Drug Administration, by the end of April 2020, had issued upward of 90 warning letters to operators in 26 states and 11 countries, accusing them of promoting dubious elixirs and treatment programs" (Lucas, 2020).

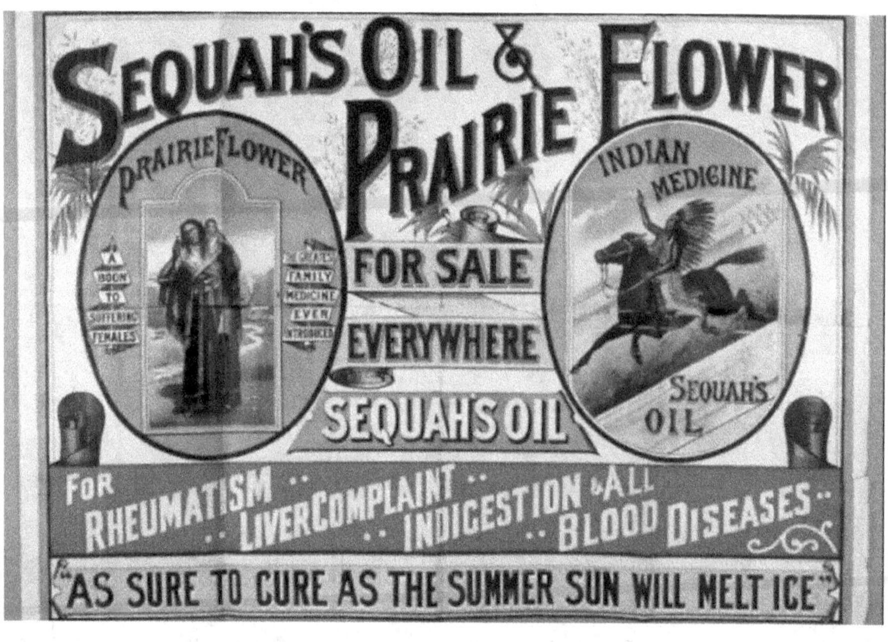

THE FOOD, DRUG, AND COSMETIC ACT OF 1938

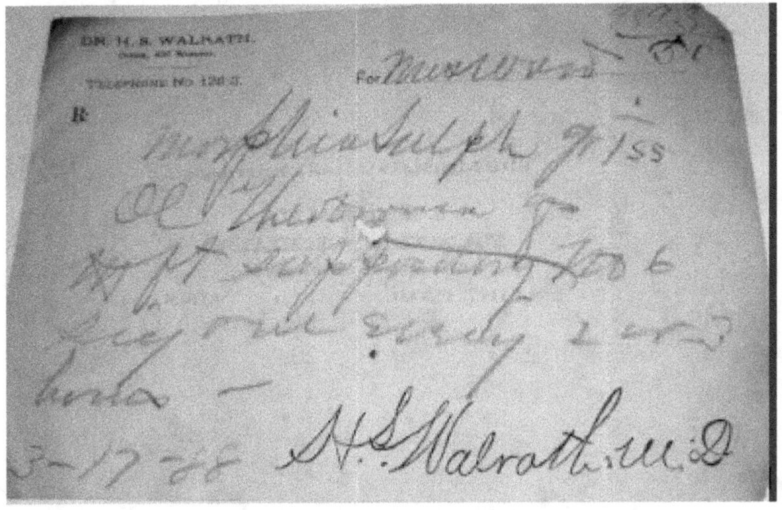

1888 prescription for morphine sulfate

FDA provides doctors and patients with the information they need to use medications wisely and ensures that drugs, both brand-name and generic, work correctly and that their health benefits outweigh their known risks. FDA's Center for Drug Evaluation and Research (CDER) is a consumer watchdog that evaluates new drugs before they come to market. While the center does not actually test the drugs itself, it does conduct limited research in the areas of drug quality, safety, and effectiveness standards. When the clinical studies have been completed and a medicine's benefits outweigh its *known* risks, FDA considers it safe enough to approve. Note the emphasis on the word "known." One must appreciate that each of us is an individual person with his or her own peculiar physiological variances in genetic makeup. The same drug that was safe and effective in the relatively small patient sample population used in clinical trials might present a problem for a patient who has an unusual sensitivity to it, resulting in an idiosyncratic drug reaction or a previously undetected side effect that was not observed in the clinical studies. In fact, most issues that arise with newly approved drugs present themselves after the drug has gone to market. This is why FDA conducts postmarketing surveillance and has set up the MedWatch program. MedWatch is the FDA Safety Information and Adverse Events Reporting System. MedWatch is the gateway for the dissemination of clinically important safety information and the reporting of serious problems with human medical products; it encourages health care professionals and patients to report all medication misadventures so that they can be documented, compiled, reviewed, verified, and added to the package inserts and medication guides (FDA, 2018).

There will always be emergency room visits due to adverse drug events. There will always be hospital admissions due to adverse drug events, and there will always be deaths due to adverse drug events. All of the above will still occur, even if every health care professional and every patient does everything correctly. In some patients, adverse drug events may be idiosyncratic and not predictable or preventable. But with careful scrutiny of patient drug allergies and a thorough medical history, adverse drug events can often be minimized.

Package inserts are generally used as reference materials by physicians and pharmacists, while medication guides are distributed directly to the patients upon filling their prescriptions. MedWatch can be accessed via FDA's website at www.fda.gov.

Once a drug is approved and comes to market, doctors must decide whether or not to prescribe a particular drug for a particular patient on an individual basis by weighing the potential benefits of the drug against any known potential risks. Even when every step in the prescribing, dispensing, and administration of a prescription is followed perfectly, drugs will have side effects. We cannot prevent all side effects, but we can try to predict them based on the published literature and based on each patient's genetic predisposition and medical history. We can be prepared to recognize common side effects so that we can discontinue a drug before significant harm is done to the patient. The package insert of each pharmaceutical product lists the frequency of various side effects. The job of the health care team is to learn and understand this information and to determine if the benefits of taking the prescription drugs outweigh any potential side effects. Pharmacists are equipped with computer programs, cell phone apps, and traditional reference books to check and cross-check drug information.

THE DRUG-APPROVAL PROCESS

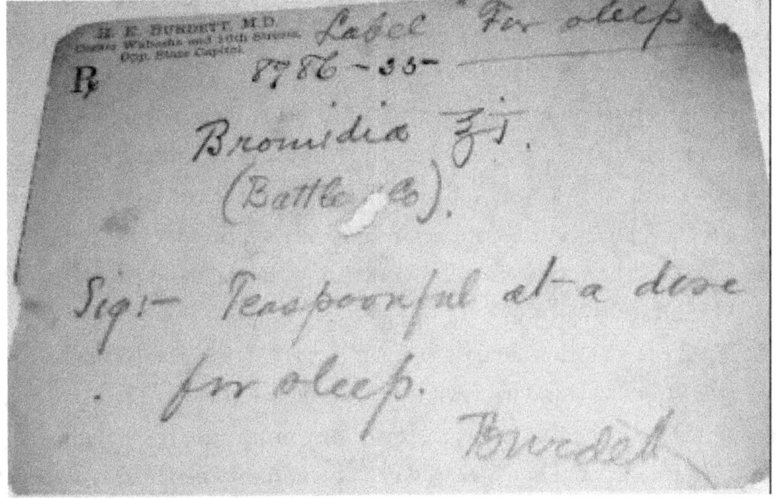

Drugs include, among other things, articles intended for use in preventing, diagnosing, curing, mitigating, or treating a disease and include components of those articles. An active pharmaceutical ingredient includes, among other things, any component that is intended to provide pharmacological activity or other direct effect in the diagnosis, cure, mitigation, treatment or prevention of disease (FDA; GAO-11-936T). The United States has the most rigorous drug-development and approval process in the world. It is estimated that it costs Big Pharma $2.5 billion to get one medication from the drawing board, to the laboratory, to the pharmacy, and, ultimately, to your medicine cabinet. This figure represents a 145 percent increase over the 2003 estimate by the Tufts Center for the Study of Drug Development (Mullin, 2014).

The mission of FDA's Center for Drug Evaluation and Research (CDER) is to ensure that drugs marketed in this country are safe and effective. The CDER does not test drugs, although the center's Office of Testing and Research does conduct limited research in the areas of drug quality, safety, and effectiveness (Hutt & Merrill, 2007). The CDER is the largest of FDA's six centers. It has responsibility for both prescription and nonprescription or over-the-counter (OTC) drugs. CDER activities include evaluating performance of drug reviews and postmarketing risk assessment of already-approved drugs to improve the health of people in the United States. The other five FDA centers have responsibility for medical and radiological devices, food and cosmetics, biologics, veterinary drugs, and tobacco products.

Some companies submit a new drug application (NDA) to introduce a new drug product into the US market. It is the responsibility of the company seeking to market a drug to test it and submit evidence that it is safe and effective. A team of CDER physicians, statisticians, chemists, pharmacologists, and other scientists reviews the sponsor's NDA containing the data and proposed labeling (Hutt & Merrill, 2007).

The 1992 Prescription Drug User Fee Act (PDUFA) established a two-tier system consisting of a standard review and a priority review. The standard FDA review applies to drugs that offer, at most, only minor improvement over existing marketed therapies. The 2002 PDUFA amendments established a ten-month goal for a standard review. The priority review designation is given to drugs that offer major advances in treatment or provide treatments where none existed. The timeline for completing a priority review is six months.

Developing a New Drug and Bringing It to Market

The discovery of a chemical compound or biological agent that shows promise as a treatment for some disease, illness, or other medical or physical condition is always an exciting phenomenon. Before clinical (human) testing is permitted to begin on an investigational new drug, substantial nonclinical testing is necessary. Researchers must show that this compound performs at the molecular level, thus indicating that it may be beneficial in treating the target condition in the human population.

In order for the drug to be tested, it must first be synthesized and purified into an active pharmaceutical ingredient (API). The FDA website explains that the research process is lengthy, complicated, and expensive, and there is no guarantee of success. Scientists often have to create and sort through hundreds or thousands of potential compounds before discovering the one that achieves a desirable result. There is no template or standard route by which drugs are developed. Pharmaceutical firms may choose to develop a drug that targets a specific disease or medical condition. Computers are helpful because they can perform three-dimensional simulations of potential chemical compounds as well as design structures that might work against it (Hutt & Merrill, 2007).

The drug can be tested in animals. The purpose of this testing is to show that, at least for animals, the drug seems to be fairly safe and appears to be effective in treating the target condition (or something similar to it). Next, scientists test the drug in humans. This testing entails a set of logical steps to establish the largest dose that a person can tolerate, to find the dose (or a couple of doses) that seems to offer the best combination of safety and efficacy, and to demonstrate convincingly that the drug works. There is also continuous monitoring of the safety of the drug in the ever-increasing number of users after it is approved and marketed (Hutt & Merrill, 2007).

Preclinical Studies: Do No Harm

Before any proposed treatment can be tested on humans, there must be at least some reason to believe that the treatment might work and that it will not put the subjects at undue risk. Thus, every promising chemical compound or biological agent must undergo an investigational new drug (IND) period during which a series of tests is run to assemble this body of evidence before the drug is ever given to a human subject. These "before-human" experiments are called preclinical studies, and they're carried out in a progressive sequence:

theoretical molecular studies

chemical studies

studies on cells and tissues

animal studies

In 1960 Dr. Frances Kelsey was hired by FDA in Washington, DC. At that time, the drug Kevadon (thalidomide) had already been approved in Canada, Europe, and Africa as a painkiller and tranquilizer that was used to alleviate morning sickness in pregnant women. Naturally, the manufacturer of Kevadon, Richardson Merrell, was persistent in trying to get the drug into the US market. Kelsey had concerns about the drug's safety and demanded more testing, citing an English study that documented side effects from the drug. Kelsey was eventually hailed as a hero when researchers discovered that thalidomide crosses the placental barrier and was at fault for birth defects in European infants whose mothers had taken the drug during pregnancy. Her work led to drug-testing reforms requiring stricter limits on the testing and distribution of new drugs. In 1962 Kelsey received the President's Award for Distinguished Federal Civilian Service from President John F. Kennedy.

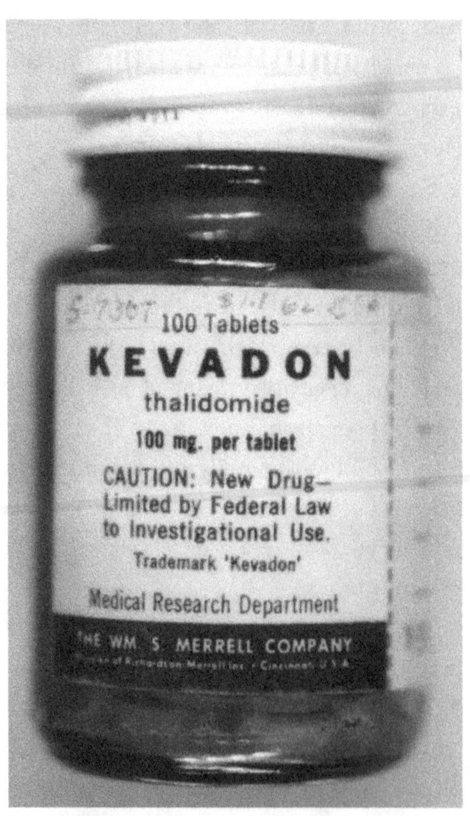

Phase 1 Clinical Trial: Determining the Maximum Tolerated Dose

The age-old saying that the "dose makes the poison" implies that any substance can be lethal in sufficiently large doses. Phase 1 trials are typically conducted on healthy human volunteers without the disease or condition being considered for treatment. Phase 1 trials are designed to determine safety and represent the first step in human drug testing. The goal is to determine how much drug you can safely give a person while minimizing dose-limiting toxicities (DLTs). The first phase 1 trial usually involves single dosing; others may involve repetitive dosing patterns to replicate the drug regimen that will actually be administered to patients. The dose of the drug is gradually increased to see if the drug becomes toxic at higher levels or if any possible side effects appear. These preliminary drug trials are usually small, containing about twenty to one hundred participants (Hutt & Merrill, 2007).

Phase 2 Clinical Trial: Exploring the Drug's Performance

Upon completion of the phase 1 studies, researchers will have an idea of the maximum tolerated dose for the drug. Then they must determine the drug's safety and efficacy at various doses in patients who have the disease or condition to be treated or cured. Factors that must be considered include the route of administration (oral, sublingual, intravenous, topical, etc.), frequency of administration, and duration of therapy. Before and after drug administration, data are gathered relating to the safety and efficacy of the drug. The goal is to determine what dose provides the highest efficacy with the fewest safety problems. This phase can last from a few months to a few years. Fewer than half these drugs will progress to the next clinical research phase (Hutt & Merrill, 2007).

Phase 3: Proving That the Drug Works

Phase 3 represents the final phase of clinical testing and involves from three hundred to three thousand patients who have the disease or condition. Safety and efficacy are monitored. During this period, researchers work with FDA to test the drug's most appropriate dosage, patient population, and other factors that determine whether the drug is approvable.

After a pharmaceutical company has completed its collection and analysis of all the data from the clinical trials and can prove that a drug is safe and effective in treating a condition, it submits a new-drug application (NDA) to FDA. The application includes clinical trial data, preclinical information, labeling information, details on the drug's manufacturing process, drug-abuse potential, and directions for patient use. If FDA accepts the NDA for review, the agency has between six and ten months to approve or disprove the drug. FDA has the authority to hold an advisory board meeting, enlisting outside experts to assess the pharmaceutical manufacturer's data and recommend whether to approve the drug. Sometimes there are concerns that must be resolved before approval; the reviewer may request additional data before making a final decision. In addition to reviewing the application, FDA also inspects the clinical study sites. If the drug is not approved, FDA will provide the drugmaker with a complete response letter stating why the drug was not approved and what procedures to follow before resubmitting the application for approval (Hutt & Merrill, 2007).

Postmarketing Surveillance—Keeping an Eye on the Marketed Drug

When the clinical studies showing safety and efficacy have been completed, and a medicine's benefits have been determined to outweigh its known risks, FDA considers it safe enough to approve (Hutt & Merrill, 2007).

Even after a drug has been approved for sale, FDA constantly monitors potential safety problems with marketed medicines. Adverse drug reactions represent a broad spectrum of severity and impact on public health. Postmarketing surveillance of the general population often brings new side effects and drug interactions to light that were not detected during the clinical trials, which typically represent a significantly smaller pool of patients (Hutt & Merrill, 2007).

Usually, a benefit-risk reassessment is prompted by the appearance of a particular sign, symptom, symptom complex, or diagnosis. A drug may be used for prevention, prophylaxis, or treatment of a particular disorder. On certain occasions, a drug may be necessary for a life-threatening condition. The acceptable risk for a drug used to save someone's life will undoubtedly be higher. For example, when an individual is suffering an anaphylactic allergic reaction due to a nut allergy or a bee sting, he or she is going to reach for epinephrine. Epinephrine injections work to counteract the symptoms of anaphylaxis by opening the airways to reduce breathing difficulties, narrow the blood vessels to combat low blood pressure, and case feelings of faintness (Goodman et al., 1990). Does epinephrine have side effects? Yes, it does. The most common side effects may include increase in heart rate, stronger or irregular heartbeat, sweating, nausea and vomiting, difficulty breathing, paleness, dizziness, weakness or shakiness, headache, apprehension, nervousness, or anxiety (Goodman et al, 1990). Any patient who is minutes away from death due to an allergic reaction will tell you that the benefit (staying alive) of epinephrine far outweighs any of these potential risks.

Insulin is notorious for causing side effects such as weight gain and hypoglycemia (low blood sugar). Despite these risk factors, insulin is a lifesaving necessity for all patients with type 1 diabetes. Prior to the discovery of insulin in 1921, type 1 diabetes was a death sentence. In this example, the benefit of using insulin is staying alive, which obviously trumps the risks of hypoglycemia and weight gain (ADA, 2019).

Another example is that of sleep aids. Millions of us have been using prescription sleep aids for decades. Certainly, we have been well aware of well-known risks such as residual daytime sedation, sleepwalking, sleep driving, and memory issues. A new study takes our concerns to the next level, linking sleeping pills to cancer and premature death. The British medical journal *BMJ Open* concluded that receiving hypnotic prescriptions was associated with greater than threefold increased hazards of death, even when fewer than eighteen pills per year were prescribed (Kripke, 2020). This association held separate analyses for several commonly used hypnotics and for newer shorter-acting drugs. The observed excess mortality could not be explained, even after taking into account preexisting comorbid variables such as obesity, smoking, and other poor health conditions. This is a classic example of a benefit-versus-risk scenario. I am not a physician, but I do not think that insomnia is typically considered a life-threatening diagnosis. Sleeping pills are *not* lifesaving drugs. If there is indeed such a significantly higher risk of death from using these medications, patients must think twice about taking these drugs, and doctors must think twice about prescribing them.

MEDICAL AND MEDICATION ERRORS

Adverse Drug Reactions

Approximately 250,000 Americans die each year as a result of medical errors (Allen, M., 2016). Another 128,000 Americans die each year as a result of taking prescription medicines as prescribed. These numbers do not include those people killed by overdosing on prescription painkillers and heroin (Schroeder, 2016).

These figures can be minimized and mitigated by proper screenings at the prescriber and pharmacy levels. It's up to the patient, prescriber, and pharmacist to determine whether the benefit of taking a particular medication outweighs any known risks of adverse drug events. Prescribers can ask patients appropriate questions to determine whether they are good candidates for particular medications.

Pharmacists can screen computerized patient profiles to identify any potential drug interactions that may occur by adding a new drug to the regimen. Community pharmacists are in the best position to prevent and recognize adverse drug reactions. Major problems occur when patients use multiple prescribers and multiple pharmacies because there is often no continuity of care and no communication between the various prescribers and pharmacies. Polypharmacy, including duplications of therapy, are common culprits of drug interactions that result in falls, emergency department visits, hospital admissions, and deaths. In the geriatric population, falls are the leading cause of injuries and deaths from injuries. From a public health perspective, falls are a major cause of morbidity and mortality. From a consultant pharmacist's perspective, a significant number of these falls may be attributed to medication misadventures.

Side Effects

Even when every step in the prescribing, dispensing, and administration of a prescription is followed perfectly, there will always be some percentage of patients that suffer side effects. Common side effects with many drugs include nausea, vomiting, diarrhea, and constipation, as these medications pass through our digestive system and get absorbed into the systemic circulation. Often, side effects can be alleviated by simple measures such as taking the medication with a meal or snack. For example, the nonsteroidal anti-inflammatory drug (NSAID) ibuprofen, the active ingredient in Advil and Motrin, is best taken with food or milk to avoid such side effects.

For other drugs, the opposite holds true. The drug Fosamax, used for osteoporosis, comes with specific warnings to take it first thing in the morning on a completely empty stomach. Dizziness and drowsiness are also common side effects with many categories of medications, including antidepressants, muscle relaxants, blood pressure medications, diabetes medications, and pain medications. This is of particular concern in the elderly, who are more susceptible to falls and who, by definition, already suffer from compromised liver and kidney function. Decreased metabolism by the liver and impaired elimination by the kidneys often result in dangerous and potentially deadly drug accumulation in our seniors. Of particular clinical importance is a parameter known as creatinine clearance. Creatinine clearance and the associated glomerular filtration rate (GFR) measure the functionality of the kidneys. Often, side effects can be prevented by using a lower dose of a drug, allowing for longer intervals between doses, or switching to a different drug. When it comes to drug dosing and titration, the best advice is to *start low and go slow*. Even over-the-counter medications can prove harmful, especially in the elderly. Diphenhydramine, the active ingredient in Benadryl, is a very potent and sedating antihistamine indicated for allergies. While the 50 mg dose requires a prescription, the 25 mg version is available as an over-the-counter product. Many people, including seniors, take diphenhydramine "off-label" as a sleeping pill. Not only does diphenhydramine cause significant residual sedation the following morning, it can also contribute to falls if the patient wakes up in the middle of the night to use the bathroom.

Certain diabetes medications, insulin in particular, can lower blood glucose faster than a patient might have anticipated, throwing him or her into an unpredictable state of hypoglycemia (low blood glucose). Hypoglycemia is a medical emergency that requires immediate administration of glucose. If not treated promptly, the patient may begin to have seizures and go into a state of unconsciousness, possibly resulting in death. A quick way to save someone from hypoglycemia is to offer them a cupful of orange juice or other sugary drink. If possible, check their blood sugar and remain with them (call 911 if necessary) until they recover completely, and then encourage them to have a snack or a meal (ADA, 2020). All caregivers should be trained in basic diabetes management, not only for the health and well-being of the individuals that they care for but also because we are all at risk for diabetes and should be familiar with the constructs of primary, secondary, and tertiary prevention.

Psychotropic medications such as clozapine, ziprasidone, risperidone, and others, for example, are notorious for inducing metabolic abnormalities, including diabetes, in otherwise healthy patients. It is commonplace for a previously physically healthy individual to find himself or herself checking blood glucose. These same drugs can also induce a pseudo-Parkinsonism, manifested by uncontrollable body movements. But these drugs also increase the quality of life for the patients who use them. Individuals who otherwise might not be able to hold down jobs or raise families are able to do all these things. When it comes to prescribing medications, we must weigh the potential therapeutic benefits against the possible risks for adverse drug events. Always start with the lowest-possible dose in order to minimize any intolerable side effects. We can't necessarily prevent ADRs and side effects, but we can try to predict them based on the published literature and each patient's predisposition and medical history. We can be prepared to recognize common side effects so that we can discontinue a drug before significant harm is done to the patient.

The manufacturer's package insert of each pharmaceutical product lists the frequency of various side effects. The expertise of the pharmacist is to read, interpret, and apply this information clinically in order to determine whether the benefits of taking the prescription drugs outweigh any potential side effects. Until proven otherwise, a good pharmacist will instinctively suspect medications as the potential culprit in any adverse event that may present itself.

Patients and caregivers are also involved in the decision-making process. Only when the benefits clearly outweigh the risks should a patient take a prescription medication. Never should a patient be forced or coerced into taking a medication he or she does not feel comfortable taking. Even hospitalized patients have the right to refuse any or all medications. Again, the purpose of this book is not to turn patients away from taking lifesaving medications. As patients, many of us will need to take at least some medications at certain points in our lives in order to thrive and survive. We should all understand that in most cases, most of us should take our medications as prescribed. Still, every patient needs to be treated as a unique human being, and prescribers must always weigh the benefits and risks of each medication before deciding which medications are best suited for each individual patient. In general, the fewer total medications one takes, the fewer the risks of side effects and drug interactions. The pharmacist can help patients weigh the risks and benefits of taking each particular medication. By trivializing the importance of the pharmacist or by not including a pharmacist on the team, we take away the safety net, and we significantly compromise patient safety. With the rise of hospitalists who do not know their patients and the decline of traditional patient-doctor and patient-pharmacist relationships, Americans are pretty much on their own when it comes to understanding their medications.

Narrow Therapeutic Index Drugs

Most common drugs are relatively safe at various dosage levels. Ibuprofen, for example, can be taken at doses between 200 mg and 800 mg per dose. Certainly, the risk of side effects increases as the dosage increases, but many people can and do take doses as low as 200 mg and as high as 800 mg. Penicillin, as long as you are not allergic to it, is another example of a drug that is safe in doses ranging from 250 mg up to ten times that much. High doses of penicillin and amoxicillin are routinely used as prophylaxis before dental visits. But narrow therapeutic index (NTI) drugs are much more dangerous in overdose or underdosing. Even a fractional deviation from the recipe can have disastrous consequences. A drug with an NTI has a very small difference between toxic and therapeutic doses (Goodman et al., 1990).

Let's look at an NTI drug such as Coumadin. Generically known as warfarin, this drug is a highly potent anticoagulant. Introduced in 1948 (unbelievably), it was and still is used as a pesticide against rodents, causing them to bleed out after ingestion. In the early 1950s, it was studied and found to be relatively safe and effective in preventing the abnormal formation and migration of blood clots. The window of safety of this drug is very narrow, with no margin for error. Very small variations in the dosage can have dramatic therapeutic or toxic effects. Too low a dose, and the patient can get a blood clot. Too high a dose, and uncontrollable bleeding can occur, leading to a horrible death. My fear is that an imported lot of uninspected Chinese- or Indian-manufactured warfarin could (accidentally or intentionally) be subpotent or superpotent, causing strokes, heart attacks, or massive uncontrolled bleeding.

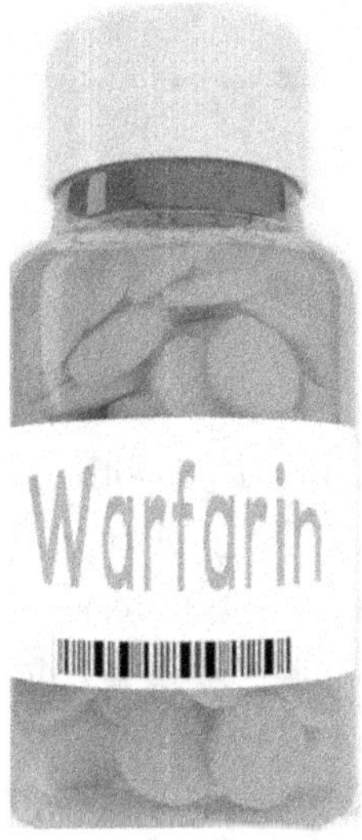

Made in China

It is unlikely that the FDA would ever have been given the opportunity to assay this particular batch of this extremely dangerous blood thinner. Soon enough, hundreds or thousands of unsuspecting patients would have been bleeding out along Main Street, USA. Who knows how long it would have taken or how many people would have died before it was determined that the tainted drug was the culprit? The only way to avoid the potential catastrophic bloodbath associated with a "Warfarin Day" is to mandate that all NTI be manufactured on US soil under the protective cloak of the FDA. Every single batch of every NTI drug should be assayed in a United States–based pharmaceutical laboratory for bioequivalence before being released for distribution. There is no other way to guarantee the safety of the American public.

Recalls, Market Withdrawals, & Safety Alerts

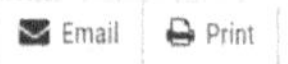

The list below provides information gathered from press releases and other public notices about certain recalls of FDA-regulated products. Not all recalls have press releases or are posted on this page. See Additional information about recalls for a more complete listing.

Other NTI drugs include lithium, levothyroxine, phenytoin, and digoxin. Small changes in doses of these drugs often manifest with very large fluctuations in blood levels and can be harmful or deadly in overdosage (Goodman et al., 1990). The best rule of thumb when dosing an NTI drug is to start low and go slow. We can always increase the dose if necessary, but we cannot retrieve a dose once we give too much. If the drug is tainted with an impurity, then it may be subpotent or superpotent and may behave unpredictably. Based on the huge volume of uninspected, counterfeit foreign drugs entering our supply chain, this prescription for disaster is continuing to manifest again and again. "Nearly 100,000 people die every year either because they are poisoned by bad ingredients in counterfeit drugs or because the counterfeit doesn't treat their illness" (the Center for Safe Internet Pharmacies, 2014). All the while, American citizens continue to seek drugs from anonymous overseas sources.

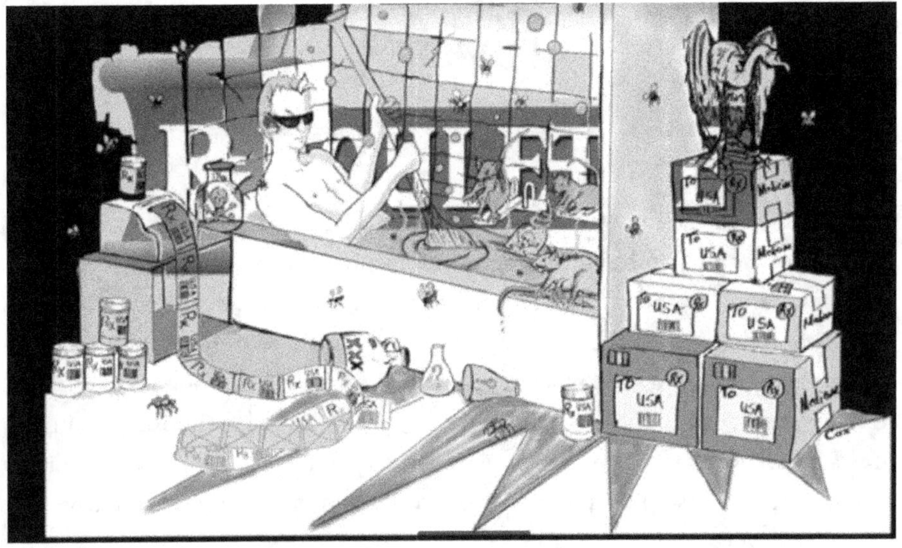

Guy in his bathtub with an oar, mixing your drugs (artist: Shelly J. Cox)

Other counterfeit drugs identified by FDA include Botox, Cialis, and the chemotherapy drug BiCNU. BiCNU is used to treat certain types of brain cancer, multiple myeloma, and lymphoma (Hodgkin's and non-Hodgkin's). According to FDA (2015), "Counterfeit Botox was found in the United States drug supply chain and may have been sold to doctors' offices and medical clinics nationwide." FDA cannot confirm that the manufacturing, quality assurance, storage conditions, and handling of these suspect products follow US standards. The reader can visit the following FDA website for additional information:

http://www.fda.gov/drugs/drugsafety/ucm443217.htm

Consumers who unwittingly purchase substandard prescription medications online are simply gambling, buying random pills that will arrive from some unknown faraway land. By definition, these knockoffs are deemed adulterated and misbranded if they are not FDA approved. In all probability, they will be counterfeit, containing too little or too much of the intended active ingredient. In some cases, they will be harmful or deadly. Those who choose to spin the prescription roulette wheel are gambling with their lives. Please do not order drugs online. Please question your mail-order pharmacy and ask them where your drugs were made.

IMPORTED DRUGS: THE GREAT GENERIC FRAUD

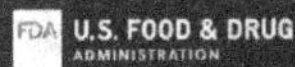

← Home / Drugs / Drug Safety and Availability / Counterfeit Versions of Cialis tablets identified entering the United States

Counterfeit Versions of Cialis tablets identified entering the United States

f Share   Tweet   in Linkedin   Email   Print

Drug Safety and Availability

FDA Updates and Press Announcements on NDMA in Zantac (ranitidine)

Information about Nitrosamine Impurities in Medications

FDA is alerting consumers and health care professionals that counterfeit versions of Cialis 20 mg tablets were found in the mail on its way to a U.S. consumer. While this shipment was stopped, FDA is concerned about other possible mail shipments to consumers. FDA laboratory analysis showed the counterfeit versions contain multiple active ingredients, which if used could result in adverse effects or harm. Consumers should only buy prescription medicines from state-licensed pharmacies located in the U.S.

FDA cannot confirm that the manufacturing, quality, storage, and handling of these products follow U.S. standards because these products are from an unknown source. Therefore, these products are considered unsafe and should not be used.

Canada's good manufacturing practices mirror those of the United States. But just because drugs may appear to have been shipped to the United States from our neighbor to the north, there is no guarantee that those products were manufactured there. Transshipment is the shipment of drugs to one destination to obscure their source and disguise their products from customs and then immediately reshipping to another destination (Partnership for Safe Medications). "Canadian" medications are often imposters, manufactured in uninspected facilities and fetid basements across all corners of the globe, only to eventually find their way into Canadian warehouses and pharmacies. Often these counterfeits are immediately reshipped to the United States without ever entering the Canadian drug supply. These drugs are *never inspected* by Canadian or US authorities. China, the epicenter of the coronavirus, loves to flood the global marketplace with toxic pharmaceuticals. From China, these nonbioequivalent products often travel through the

Middle East and Europe, changing hands more than thirty times before reaching buyers in Canada and the United States (Lewis, 2009). Vomiting, diarrhea, abdominal pain, joint pain, hair loss, blurry vision, dizziness, respiratory problems, nervous system disruption, coma, and death have all occurred upon ingestion of these poisoned, transshipped knockoffs that have never been inspected. Even if the product that you ingest contains no poisons or wrong medications, a potentially lifesaving medication without active ingredient will cause harm and potentially death. Many counterfeits contain only dextrose, lactose, starch, salt, and other inert fillers that might not be poisons in and among themselves but deprive sick patients of the treatments and cures they are depending on. Drug counterfeiters are literally getting away with murder every time an innocent patient spins the roulette wheel and falls victim to adulterated and misbranded imported pharmaceutical fakes.

Just as Samuel Hopkins Adams described patent medicines as "the Great American Fraud," so have imported nonbioequivalent drugs become "the Great Generic Fraud."

Another prime example of deadly knockoffs can be found in the counterfeit Avastin case mentioned previously. While the original source remains unknown, the fake drug traveled through Turkey, Switzerland, Denmark, and the United Kingdom before being imported by a Canada Drugs–contracted middleman distributor in Tennessee. The Avastin scandal was revisited in this recent documentary on counterfeit Canadian medications:

https://www.abcactionnews.com/money/consumer/taking-action-for-you/
popular-online-canadian-pharmacy-ordered-to-shutdown-over-counterfeit-medicine

Canada Drugs opened a Bangalore-based company so it could purchase drugs directly from manufacturers in India, circumventing the safety net of FDA.

History repeats itself. The Federal Food, Drug, and Cosmetic of Act 1938 was enacted for a reason. The complexity of the drug supply chain, the tsunami of imported drugs, and the overwhelming number of foreign drug establishments (purchasing raw materials from unknown sources) producing these drugs make it nearly impossible for FDA, with limited resources, to properly protect all of us. The probability of one or more injurious raw materials entering the supply chain during the manufacturing, preparation, propagation, compounding, or processing of a drug and finding their way into the finished drug products sitting on the shelves in our very own medicine cabinets is very high. Here is a great link to an FDA webpage describing supply-chain integrity:

https://www.fda.gov/Drugs/DrugSafety/DrugIntegrityandSupplyChainSecurity/default.htm

Despite all the examples proving unequivocally that the importation of foreign drug ingredients and finished drug products has already proved deadly, a recent Kaiser Family Foundation poll showed that the majority of Americans actually approve of such importation. A direct link to the information can be accessed here:

https://www.kff.org/health-costs/press-release/poll-majorities-of-democrats-republicans-and-independents-support-actions-to-lower-drug-costs-including-allowing-americans-to-buy-drugs-from-canada/.

We have some states (including Colorado, Florida, Maine, and Vermont) that are seeking to circumvent the protections afforded by the Food, Drug, and Cosmetic Act by permitting the importation of cheap foreign drugs from Canada and other countries. The momentum for drug importation is growing at the state and federal level. It is totally understandable and commendable that these states and the president want to save their constituents money on their prescriptions. Regrettably, the passage of such legislation would immediately open up a Pandora's box of low-grade drugs that would quickly flow across our borders, plunging us back into the unregulated days before we had the protection of FDA.

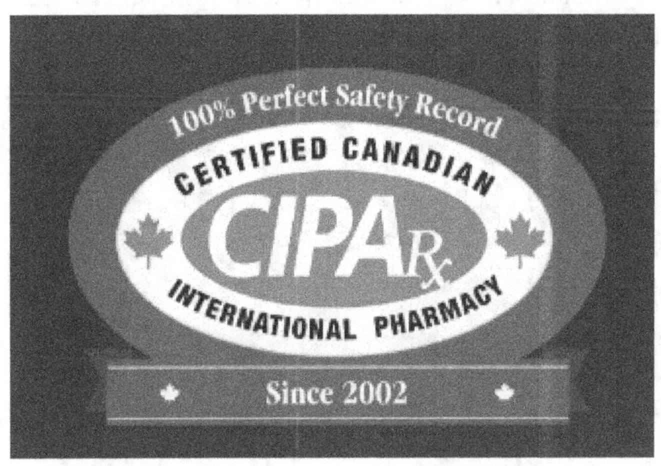

"Canadian" drugs have not been inspected by the FDA and may be counterfeits manufactured in China or India in someone's filthy bathtub.

The politicians who are advocating for imported drugs are good people who want to help our senior citizens and working-class persons to be able to afford their life-sustaining prescription medications. Yet instead they are circumventing the protective cloak of FDA and are placing their constituents in harm's way. The death toll that would result from consumption of these cheaper toxic drug products would be many times worse than the current COVID-19 disaster. US citizens will drop like flies as they ingest innumerable nonbioequivalent medications from abroad. Visit canadadrugs.com, and you will find that the domain has been seized by FDA due to the plethora of filthy counterfeit drugs that have *already* caused the deaths of countless Americans. Phony drugs have become a major cause of treatment failures, leading to excessive morbidity (disability) and mortality (death). Furthermore, charlatan drugs have been implicated globally in contributing to the development of drug-resistant organisms in many infectious diseases of public health importance, such as tuberculosis, malaria and HIV/AIDS (Tadeg & Berhane, 2012). According to Reuters, "The human cost can be high. Low-quality and fake antimalarial drugs accounted for more than a third of samples analyzed in sub-Saharan Africa, according to a study in the *Lancet Infectious Diseases* journal. Separate research in the journal *Research and Reports in*

Tropical Medicine found Chinese-made drugs to treat malaria and other common tropical infections performed particularly poorly in tests" (Lee, 2012).

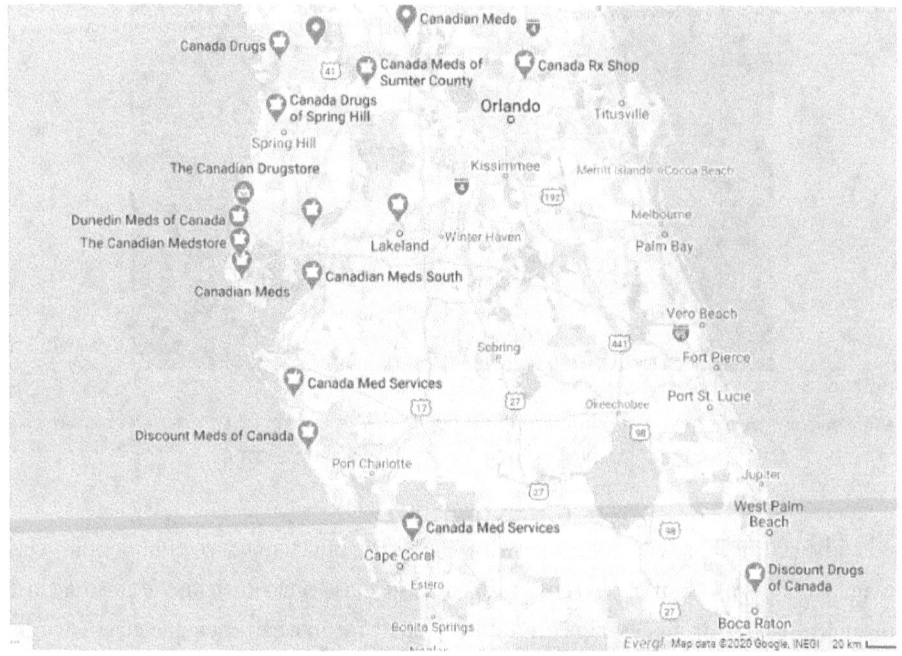

Results of Google search for "Canadian" pharmacies in Florida

The discount "Canadian" pharmacies in Florida strip malls are simply middlemen storefronts, also known as facilitators, that never take possession of the actual medications. There are no registered pharmacists on duty there, and they have no clue as to the actual source of the raw materials and finished drug products. These facilitators deal with pharmacies and suppliers located all over the globe, not just in Canada. If you think your drugs are actually shipping from Canada, think again (Levitt, 2017). On February 26, 2019, FDA issued a warning letter to CanaRx, an online Canadian pharmacy. CanaRx was cited for causing the introduction of unapproved and misbranded drugs into interstate commerce. According to FDA, "CanaRx operates as a prescription drug provider that engages in activities to cause the introduction of unapproved drugs from foreign sources into the United States in violation of the FD&C Act. Because these products are intended for use in the diagnosis, cure, mitigation, treatment, or prevention of disease and/or affect the structure or function of the body, these products are *drugs*…These products are also *new drugs* because they are not generally recognized as safe and effective for their labeled uses. New drugs may not be introduced or delivered for introduction into interstate commerce without prior approval from FDA" (Hutt & Merrill, 2007). Here is a link to an FDA press release regarding this urgent matter:

https://www.fda.gov/NewsEvents/Newsroom/PressAnnouncements/ucm632360.htm

WARNING LETTER

The United States (U.S.) Food and Drug Administration (FDA) recently reviewed your websites listed at the bottom of this letter and determined that you and your affiliates cause the introduction of unapproved new drugs and misbranded drugs into interstate commerce in violation of sections 301(a), 301(d), and 505(a) of the Federal Food, Drug, and Cosmetic Act (FD&C Act) [21 U.S.C. §§ 331(a), 331(d), and 355(a)]. While this letter refers to CanaRx Services Inc/CRX Intl (hereinafter CanaRx), the violations discussed apply to all entities conducting business by or on behalf of CanaRx. FDA requests that you immediately cease causing the distribution of violative drugs to U.S. consumers.

UNAPPROVED NEW DRUGS

CanaRx operates as a prescription drug provider that engages in activities to cause the introduction of unapproved new drugs from foreign sources into the United States in violation of the FD&C Act. Because these products are intended for use in the diagnosis, cure, mitigation, treatment, or prevention of disease and/or affect the structure or function of the body, these products are drugs within the meaning of section 201(g)(1) of the FD&C Act [21 U.S.C. § 321(g)(1)]. These products are also new drugs as defined by section 201(p) of the FD&C Act [21 U.S.C. § 321(p)] because they are not generally recognized as safe and effective for their labeled uses. New drugs may not be introduced or delivered for introduction into interstate commerce without prior approval from FDA, as described in section 505(a) of the FD&C Act [21 U.S.C. § 355(a)]. No FDA-approved applications pursuant to section 505 of the FD&C Act [21 U.S.C. § 355] are in effect for these products. Accordingly, their introduction or delivery for introduction into interstate commerce violates sections 301(d) and 505(a) of the FD&C Act [21 U.S.C. §§ 331(d) and

The federal ban on imported drugs is not always enforced at the state level. Any clown can open a storefront in Florida or on the internet and begin to skim affiliate middlemen profits by referring naive patients to "Canadian" and other global suppliers. These storefront pharmacies are often attached to rogue international pharmacies that provide noxious pretender drugs.

Unwary seniors may believe they are purchasing legitimate drugs that were manufactured in Canada, when in fact they are often harmful knockoffs manufactured worlds away, where FDA has no jurisdiction. Perhaps there is no active ingredient at all in the product, as in the Canadian Avastin example cited earlier. In other cases, there may be superpotent doses of active ingredients. In the case of a May 2020, recall, levothyroxine, a highly potent narrow therapeutic index (NTI) drug was found to have been manufactured overseas and distributed in North America. The product was subsequently recalled for having too much of the superpotent levothyroxine API. My objective here is not necessarily to identify the company (you can google it) but to provide yet another example of nonbioequivalent, foreign-made NTI generics causing harm to Americans. *I will tell you unequivocally that if this had been warfarin instead of levothyroxine, there would have been many fatalities.* Impurities may be inadvertently or intentionally laced into the mixture, as with the deadly Chinese-made heparin atrocity. Patients may think they are saving money, when in actuality they are playing a potentially deadly game of prescription roulette, as deadly poisons accumulate in their livers and damage their kidneys. These tragic stories do not always make front-page headlines, but many people in the United States and globally continue to die as a result of consumption of these toxic fakes. China was also responsible for sickening and killing hundreds of US cats and dogs that had consumed pet foods laced with the industrial poison melamine. The same poison was later found in human food products and baby formula made in China, blamed for sickening thousands of infants and killing four. Dangerous counterfeit weight-loss products, illegally imported from China and distributed from Texas, were found to contain the drug sibutramine, notorious for causing high blood pressure, seizures, tachycardia, heart attacks, and strokes (US Immigration and Customs Enforcement, 2011).

Even with Medicare, medication co-pays and deductibles still create financial burdens for senior citizens, forcing them to seek cheaper alternatives. The "doughnut hole," for example, is a coverage gap, a window during which coverage ceases and patients must endure full out-of-pocket expenses. As such, elderly patients flock to these unapproved websites and storefronts that save them up to 70 percent over regular drugstore prices. The storefronts describe themselves as a resource for those who cannot afford to pay for their medications. While the cost savings may be real, the global source of the raw materials and active pharmaceutical ingredients remains unknown. Likewise, the ambiguous and often filthy conditions of the overseas manufacturing facilities make risk of ingesting these products not worth it. It's a crapshoot as to whether or not the cost savings are going to cost you your life. These "Canadian" storefront "pharmacies" are not pharmacies at all but middlemen, transshipping drugs that have been manufactured halfway around the world using toxic ingredients purchased at the local flea market. For more information, follow this link to FDA's policy on the importation of drugs from outside the United States:

https://www.fda.gov/ForIndustry/ImportProgram/ucm173751.htm

Fake and diverted pharmaceuticals, including antibiotics and antimalarials, have been flowing out of Asia, Europe, Africa, and the Middle East for many years. Counterfeit drugs have a drastic impact on global health and welfare. These substandard products contribute to the development of drug-resistant organisms in many infectious diseases of public health significance, including malaria, tuberculosis, and HIV/AIDS. Under the Federal Food, Drug, and Cosmetic Act, unapproved, misbranded, and adulterated drugs are prohibited from importation into the United States. But even with the deadly coronavirus stifling manufacturing and distribution, there is a continuous flow of these deadly knockoff drugs flooding the global pharmaceutical supply chain.

The volume of prescription medications for personal use coming across our borders via the mail has increased exponentially in recent years as desperate individuals, including senior citizens, can no longer afford to pay the high costs of prescription drugs in the United States. Florida is well known for pharmacy storefront facilitators that act as middlemen between Canadian and other international drugstores and the astronomical number of US senior citizens looking to save money on prescription drugs. Elderly patients must endure the risks of potentially counterfeit drugs and flock by the thousands to purchase cheaper medications from ambiguous overseas suppliers and transshippers. Patient safety frequently takes a back seat to the desire to save money. These naive seniors see a Canadian postmark and are duped into believing that their medications are manufactured in Canada. In fact, they are often dangerous imposters made in someone's makeshift basement laboratory and transshipped around the world by drug smugglers. Make no mistake: the majority of the medications that arrive on your doorstep with Canadian postmarks are not manufactured in Canada, and they are never inspected by any regulatory agency. You are spinning the roulette wheel with every potentially toxic dose you ingest.

The Federal Food, Drug, and Cosmetic Act of 1938 gives FDA authority to regulate foods, drugs, cosmetics, and medical devices. The act came about as the result of many lessons learned the hard way. Pharmaceutical disasters plagued our nation before these regulations were enacted. By permitting middlemen storefront profiteers to masquerade as licensed pharmacies and circumvent the protective shield that FDA provides to the citizens of the United States of America, we are at risk of plunging back into the days of the patent medicine era, when no one knew what potentially detrimental ingredients were contained in the remedies pitched by the snake oil salesmen. Counterfeit medications purchased from fake online pharmacies or from US sources that have purchased outside of the supply chains have been found to contain contaminants including fentanyl, mercury, aluminum, lead, cadmium, arsenic, chrome, uranium, strontium, selenium, PCBs, benzopyrenes, rat poison, boric acid, antifreeze, road paint, wall paint, brick dust, floor wax, sheet rock, paint thinner, random drugs, and no drugs at all (Partnership for Safe Medications).

In 2019 Chinese authorities discovered millions of medicine capsules made with an industrial gel containing chromium, a carcinogenic heavy metal. Kudos to China for taking action in this case. Still, this serves as a prime example of how inferior raw materials frequently become part of the recipe for the nonbioequivalent drugs that are produced and exported globally. Furthermore, "unlicensed

Chinese chemical firms advertise substances that have been pulled from Western markets due to safety concerns, such as the weight-loss treatment rimonabant which was withdrawn in Europe and was never approved in the United States." It is impossible for the FDA to trace the origin of all the raw materials that are used by overseas manufacturers. While the Chinese government does not specifically endorse this practice, it does look the other way, saying foreign companies should take responsibility for standards by buying products only from properly certified exporters (Lee, 2012).

https://www.nytimes.com/2007/05/06/world/americas/06poison.html?pagewanted=all

Organized Crime: The European Connection to Stolen and Counterfeit Drugs

The WHO mentions that profits generated by the trade in counterfeit drugs make it attractive to criminal networks. In April of 2014, the *Wall Street Journal* reported that the Italian Mafia was involved in the theft of expensive cancer drugs from hospitals and suppliers. In Italy it is evidently commonplace for multiple truckloads per month of these high-ticket pharmaceuticals to mysteriously disappear. The European Medicines Agency warned in April of 2014 that Herceptin, a very expensive cancer drug manufactured by Roche, had been stolen in Italy. The product then reappeared across Europe, diluted and rendered useless. Laboratory testing by Roche confirmed that the expensive active ingredient had actually been replaced by a cheap antibiotic, and the putrefied residue was then sold throughout the United Kingdom, Germany, and Finland. Imagine how many cancer patients received absolutely no active chemotherapy in the Herceptin infusions, not to mention possible harm or death from the substituted fake drug product. The hoodwinkers profited handsomely by selling the fake product at almost $700 per dose, as if it were the real drug. Additionally, the stolen real product was probably diluted and resold many times over to local physicians and hospitals across Europe and perhaps globally (Faucon et al., 2014).

Health Care Provider Alert: Another Counterfeit Cancer Medicine Found in United States

Counterfeit Medicine

Purchasing Unapproved Drugs Is Risky Business

[2/5/2013] The Food and Drug Administration is committed to protecting the supply chain against counterfeit and unapproved medicines that enter the United States through fraudulent sources. As part of this vigilance, FDA is alerting health care professionals that an unapproved cancer medicine distributed by a U.S. company, Medical Device King (also known as Pharmalogical), is counterfeit.

FDA lab tests have confirmed that at least one batch of a counterfeit version of Roche's Altuzan distributed in the United States contains no active ingredient.

Content current as of:
02/13/2018

FDA letter alerting providers of counterfeit medicine in the supply chain

THE GLOBAL PHARMACEUTICAL SUPPLY CHAIN

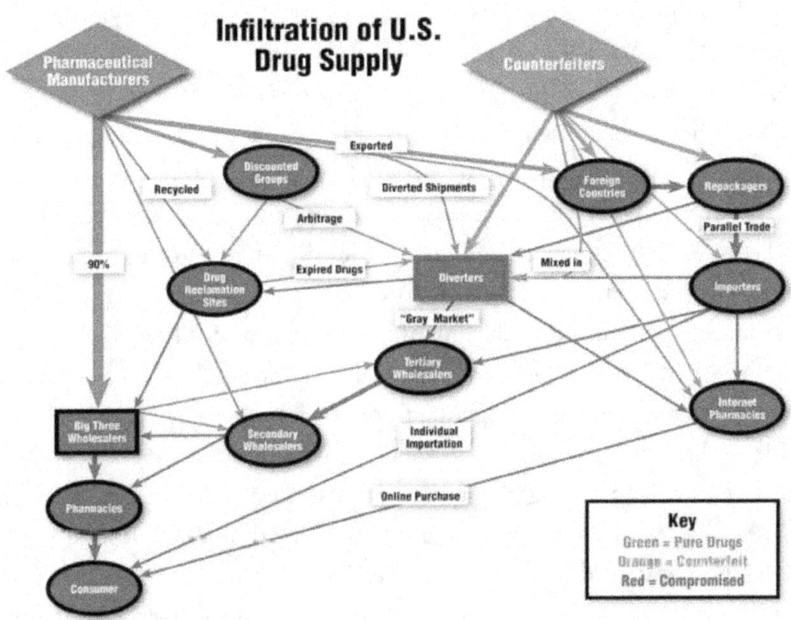

Illustration of counterfeit medicines and criminal organizations by Eric Przyswa (*Counterfeit Medications and Criminal Organisations*, by IRACM, 2013, p. 27).

Supply-Chain Integrity

How do these products appear in our medicine cabinets? We may pick them up from the corner pharmacy, but where did the pharmacist get them from? To answer these questions, one must understand the global pharmaceutical supply chain.

The pharmaceutical supply chain is the mechanism by which prescription medications begin their journey as raw materials sourced globally from all around the world and end up as finished drug products in our medicine cabinets. These raw materials include active pharmaceutical ingredients (API) as well as excipients (supposedly inert ingredients such as colors, binders, and fillers) that are blended together just like in any recipe in any cookbook but in massive quantities.

Domestically, this cookbook is governed by strict rules and regulations and is overseen by FDA. Manufacturers must adhere to strict standard operating procedures (SOPs) and good manufacturing practices (GMPs). Overseas, these standards are impossible to enforce because FDA cannot conduct unannounced inspections of the manufacturing facilities. After production, the finished pharmaceuticals are transported all around the world to wholesale distributors and then to hospitals, retail pharmacies, mail-order outlets, and other types of dispensaries. The medications are eventually dispensed to patients by the hospitals and pharmacies. In addition to the "big three" primary US wholesalers, there is also a global "gray market" of secondary and tertiary wholesalers that may inadvertently receive compromised and/or counterfeit pharmaceuticals that have slipped into the supply chain. These secondary and tertiary wholesalers then become a vector, transferring the adulterated and misbranded drugs to other wholesalers as well as to unsuspecting pharmacies and dispensaries.

Once upon a time, the supply chain was 100 percent domestic. FDA could more easily track all raw materials and finished drug products from start to finish. Today, the entire supply chain is globalized, with individual ingredients originating from every corner of the globe and eventually ending up in our medicine cabinets. Manufacturers pick and choose from suppliers, licensed and unlicensed, all over the world. *It's tantamount to a global pharma flea market for raw materials, where bargain hunters search for the cheapest price without regard to product quality or patient safety.* Click or copy this link or follow the QR code to see for yourself:

https://www.alibaba.com/showroom/alibaba-pharmaceuticals.html

Manufacturing, particularly of generic drugs, is frequently done overseas. Raw materials and completed drug products routinely come from China and India, where pharmaceutical production is grossly underregulated. When it comes to consumer safety, no one really cares. China and India provide us with many well-educated and intelligent individuals who can run intellectual circles around many Americans. As the author of this book and an advocate of global public health, I have the utmost respect and empathy for all persons on this planet. *While this book is obviously very critical of the underregulated Chinese and Indian pharmaceutical industries, it is not targeting the individual people of China or India, whom I respect very much.*

As the coronavirus rages on, and the global pharmaceutical supply chain comes to an abrupt halt, the United States is now paying the price for having given up our FDA-protected and regulated generic pharmaceutical industry to cheaper, inferior, unregulated overseas manufacturers. It is essential that Big Pharma, particularly generic firms, take advantage of the newly reduced corporate tax rate and bring drug manufacturing back home. It is a matter of national security that the integrity of our pharmaceutical supply chain is never interrupted again. *Our military consumes medications made in China. What happens when China decides to intentionally remove all API and/or add "extra" ingredients to their exported drugs?* China has plenty of troops, tanks, and missiles that are incessantly on parade, but they are not going to need them to control the world.

In many areas, sanitation is primitive, contamination is frequent, and regulation is sketchy at best. In today's global environment, when pharmacists in the United States order prescription drug products from their local wholesalers, the stock bottles often arrive labeled from manufacturers on the other side of the world, where regulations (good manufacturing practices) may or may not exist. Raw materials for the pharmaceuticals that populate the shelves in US pharmacies and the medicine cabinets of US households are often purchased via the overseas global flea market, where the FDA has no jurisdiction. Active pharmaceutical ingredients, as well as excipients, often originate from underdeveloped nations, where corruption is rampant and bribery is commonplace. Chinese chemical companies making API are selling their products on the open market with few or no checks. Historically, whichever vendor had the cheapest price for raw materials made the sale, while local inspectors were routinely paid to look the other way. CPhI is an international pharmaceutical fair where hundreds of exhibitors pay to display their pharmaceutical machinery and technology, pharmaceutical packaging, excipients, specialty chemicals, and API for sale. A quick look at the exhibitors list online (cphi-online.com) shows that some firms claim to be GMP certified while many others make no mention of GMP certification. The problem here is that "any number of pharmaceutical companies go no further than looking for API suppliers based only on price" (Lee, 2012). Vendors that are not GMP certified have lower overhead costs and cheaper prices versus those firms that spend the time and money to get GMP certified. Without vendor GMP certification, customers (pharma companies) cannot be certain of the quality of the ingredients that are being purchased. Consequently, nonbioequivalent knockoffs, often containing toxic additives such as mercury, lead, arsenic, rat poison, antifreeze, Sheetrock, road paint, and an infinite number of other potentially deadly contaminants, continue to infiltrate the global supply chain.

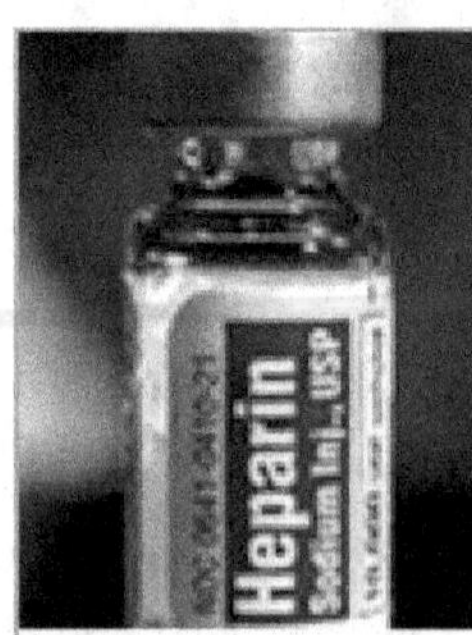

GAO-11-936T Report on Drug Safety

On September 14, 2011, testimony was given before the Committee on Health, Education, Labor and Pensions at the US Senate. The discussion focused on FDA's inspection of foreign manufacturing establishments, the information FDA had on these establishments, and recent FDA initiatives to improve its oversight of the supply chain. Some of the findings included the following:

Inspections of foreign drug manufacturers are an important element of FDA's oversight of the supply chain, but the GAO's prior work showed that FDA conducts relatively few such inspections. Additionally, FDA announces its overseas inspections weeks in advance, allowing unscrupulous manufacturers to sanitize the factories, fudge the data, and serve temporary eviction notices to the multitude of flies and rats that reside there. GAO reported that in fiscal year 2007, FDA inspected only 8 percent of foreign establishments subject to inspection. It estimated that, at that rate, it would take FDA about thirteen years to inspect all such establishments just one time each. GAO recommended that FDA increase the number of foreign inspections conducted at a frequency comparable to domestic establishments with similar characteristics. FDA subsequently increased the number of foreign establishments. FDA's inspection efforts in fiscal year 2009 represented a 27 percent increase in the number of inspections conducted when compared to fiscal year 2007—424 and 333 inspections, respectively. But FDA acknowledged that it is far from achieving foreign drug inspection rates comparable to domestic inspection rates—the agency inspected 1,015 domestic establishments in 2009 (GAO, 2011).

A recent exposé in *Bloomberg Businessweek* highlights the fact that overseas FDA inspections are on the decline once again (Edney, 2019). With thousands of overseas suppliers and factories in need of inspections and relatively few available inspectors, this means that even more contaminants and carcinogens, including the deadly NDMA, continue to enter the global supply chain and kill people. Examples are plentiful and include the countless number of worldwide product recalls of irbesartan, losartan ranitidine, metformin, and many other drugs. Quality assurance testing using HPLC (defined elsewhere in this book) would easily identify these impurities—if the tests were actually being run. Of course, without the power of the *surprise* inspection, there is ample time for foreign manufacturers to conjure up whatever data they wish. There is enough time to construct a brand-new, clean room or even a building.

Reuters' "Special Report on China's Wild East Drug Store" documented a pharma inspector who was given the runaround when visiting a factory that was immaculately clean and had many years' worth of perfect logbooks—all in the same handwriting (Lee, 2012). The necessary connecting pipes to funnel steam and waste gases out of the plant were absent. It was obvious that the drugs were not manufactured at this particular location but more likely at a noncompliant facility somewhere else. No one knows for sure because many foreign drug firms have never been FDA inspected, but it has been suggested that up to half of all foreign generic drug stability data and batch records are routinely fabricated, with absolutely no real assays actually being conducted. For example, if there is one "good" batch of drugs, those results are simply saved, copied, and reused over and over again with minor alterations in the data, so that all the batch records don't appear identical to one another. Local authorities are easily bribed, and FDA only materializes for on-site inspections every decade or so. There have been no overseas FDA pharmaceutical company inspections during the COVID-19 pandemic, even though drug manufacturing has now resumed.

Language barriers are another challenge that FDA encounters during foreign drug manufacturer inspections, with translators typically being supplied by the same entities that are being inspected. This presents an obvious conflict of interest, as inspectors are intentionally run in circles, raising serious concerns about the integrity of the translators and the accuracy of the information being supplied. Often piles of batch records and other manufacturing documents mysteriously vanish when an FDA inspector turns his or her back. Finally, upon completion of the inspection, when violations are discovered, it takes months until FDA warning letters get issued and until the American public is notified. All the while, the foreign products in question continue to be consumed by the unsuspecting American public.

All Ranitidine Products (Zantac): Press Release - FDA Requests Removal

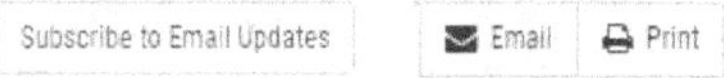

[Posted 04/01/2020]

ISSUE: The FDA announced it is requesting manufacturers to withdraw all prescription and over-the-counter (OTC) ranitidine drugs from the market immediately.

This is the latest step in an ongoing investigation of a contaminant known as N-Nitrosodimethylamine (NDMA) in ranitidine medications (commonly known by the brand name Zantac). NDMA is a probable human carcinogen (a substance that could cause cancer). FDA has determined that the impurity in some ranitidine products increases over time and when stored at higher than room temperatures may result in consumer exposure to unacceptable levels of this impurity. As a result of this immediate market withdrawal request, ranitidine products will not be available for new or existing prescriptions or OTC use in the U.S.

We are constantly bombarded with nonbioequivalent generic drugs being slipped into the supply chain with foreign, life-threatening contaminants found in their raw materials. A global recall has been underway for a countless number of blood pressure drugs, including valsartan, irbesartan, and losartan, that were produced by Chinese manufacturer Huahai and others and laced with the potentially fatal carcinogenic chemical NDMA. NDMA, a component of rocket fuel, causes cancer in animals and humans and is especially toxic to the liver. These faulty drugs were widely distributed by many generic pharma companies. In February of 2020, the FDA website reported that one of the most widely prescribed diabetes drugs, metformin, had been found to be tainted with NDMA. In May of 2020, the FDA requested that five manufacturers immediately recall their NDMA-laced nonbioequivalent versions of metformin (Sebastian, 2020). Canada, meanwhile, has recalled several generic versions of metformin for the same reason. Additionally, as of April 1, 2020, recalls have been expanded to include *all* the branded and generic prescription and over-the-counter versions of the stomach medication ranitidine (FDA, 2020). Check to make sure that your imported nonbioequivalent medications have not been recalled!

https://abcnews.go.com/Health/zantac-problem-whats-ndma/story?id=65799147

Simply put, generic drugs do not have to go through the same rigorous FDA approval process as brand-name drugs do, and Americans are dying because of this. This problem is exacerbated by the fact that the vast majority of active ingredients and excipients come from unregulated, uninspected overseas sources.

https://pittsburgh.cbslocal.com/video/3977080-blood-pressure-drug-recall-expands-again-due-to-potential-cancer-causing-chemical/

The GAO-11-936T testimony goes on to mention that "the types of inspections FDA conducts generally do not include all parts of the drug supply chain" (GAO-11-936T). Conducting inspections abroad also continues to pose unique challenges for the agency. For example, FDA faces limits on its ability to require foreign establishments to allow it to inspect their facilities. Furthermore, logistical issues preclude FDA from conducting unannounced inspections, as it does for domestic establishments. There is a huge difference in compliance when a domestic firm knows that FDA can just walk in the front door. "GAO previously reported that FDA lacked complete and accurate information on foreign drug manufacturing establishments—information necessary to understanding the supply chain. In 2008, GAO reported that FDA databases contained incorrect information about foreign establishments manufacturing drugs for the US market. FDA's lack of information hampers its ability to inspect foreign establishments. GAO recommended that FDA address these deficiencies. FDA has taken steps to do so but has not yet fully addressed GAO'S concerns" (GAO-11-936T). In the United States, Big Pharma follows good manufacturing practices (GMPs), a strict set of FDA guidelines that prevents adulterated and misbranded drugs from entering our supply chain. Conversely, there is no global regulatory body to enforce quality assurance, and foreign pharmaceutical manufacturers routinely ignore Western patents and intentionally circumvent all GMPs.

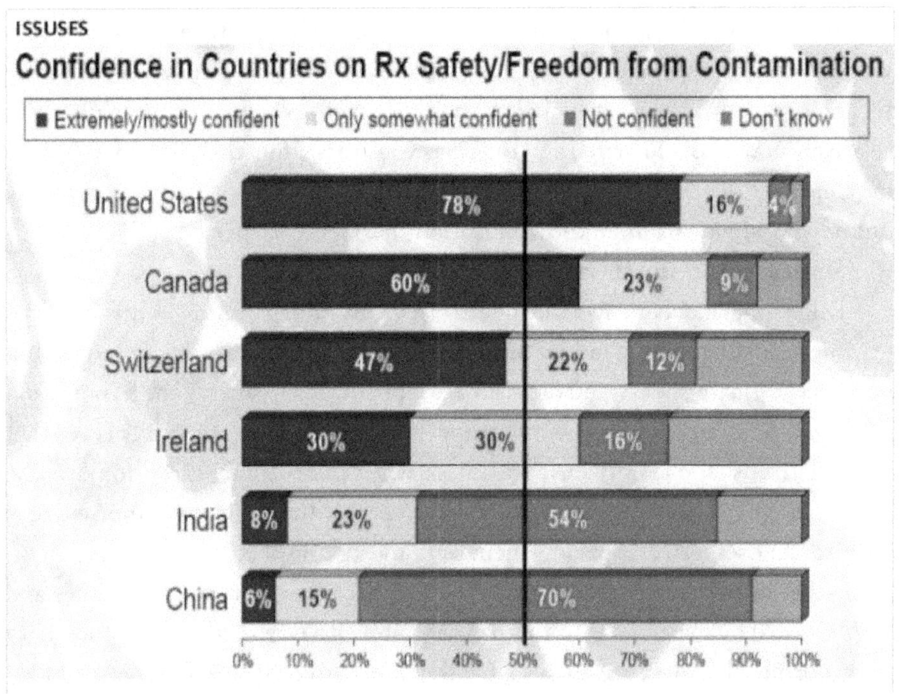

Meanwhile, even as you are reading these words, substandard foreign raw materials and finished products continue to be dispensed to US consumers. The GAO goes on to mention the following:

Given the difficulties that FDA has faced in inspecting and obtaining information on foreign drug manufacturers, and recognizing that more inspections alone are not sufficient to meet the challenges posed by globalization, the agency has begun to implement other initiatives to improve its oversight of the drug supply chain. FDA's overseas offices have engaged in a variety of activities to help ensure the safety of imported products, such as training foreign stakeholders to help enhance their understanding of FDA regulations. GAO recommended that FDA enhance its strategic and workforce planning, which FDA agreed it would do. FDA has also taken other positive steps, such as developing initiatives that would assist its oversight of products at the border, although these are not yet fully implemented. (GAO, 2011)

Perhaps the introduction of blockchain technology by Big Pharma will be helpful in tracking raw materials and finished drug products as they travel along the continuum of the global pharmaceutical chain. Manufacturers, distributors, wholesalers, pharmacies, and hospitals will be able to utilize this track and trace technology to help thwart global drug counterfeiters. This technology is still relatively new to Big Pharma, and today, as you are reading this book, *people across the world are still dropping dead* from shoddy masquerader medicines concocted by unknown individuals in unknown locations (Roberts, 2017).

Senior Citizens, Beware

Killer pharmaceuticals continue to flow into our country. All the while, organizations that have good intentions and want to save our seniors money but do not necessarily understand the risks are lobbying for legalizing the importation of drugs from Canada and certain European countries. I unequivocally agree that senior citizens (and all citizens) are at risk when they cannot afford to purchase their lifesaving drugs. It is absolutely unacceptable that so many senior citizens have to choose between paying their rent and taking their medications. I also agree that imported drugs would be cheaper because insurance companies and PBMs would be bypassed. But there is absolutely no way to guarantee the safety of imported pharmaceuticals because they circumvent the safety net of FDA. One must comprehend that although the drugs may appear to be "coming from Canada" by their postmarks, the raw materials have likely been obtained from an uncertified vendor who harvested the ingredients from the cheapest source in an unregulated environment. It's truly a crapshoot or a spin of the roulette wheel as to what random toxicity you will get. Likewise, the finished drug products may be manufactured anywhere on the globe under unknown conditions, even if they ultimately ship from Canada. I strongly encourage the reader to watch this important video on counterfeit "Canadian" drugs:

https://www.abcactionnews.com/money/consumer/taking-action-for-you/
popular-online-canadian-pharmacy-ordered-to-shutdown-over-counterfeit-medicine

In fact, these fake and potentially deadly knockoff drugs may be created in someone's dirty makeshift basement laboratory in a nonregulated environment halfway across the globe. The presence of fake drugs is even more prevalent in countries with weak drug regulation control and enforcement. Dr. Howard Zucker has warned that "countries should think about ways to make the necessary technological, legislative, and financial adjustments as quickly as possible to guarantee the availability of quality assured essential drugs" (WHO, 2006).

A good laser printer can easily produce a near-perfect phony label that the rogue drug forger simply affixes to the bottle. Despite its best efforts, FDA will not be able to protect us from these "lone-wolf" individuals, organizations, or nations that care only about profit at the expense of safety if we legalize these imports. Even today, with all the safeguards we have in place, poisoned drugs still enter the supply chain and kill us: "Counterfeit medications are part of the broader phenomenon of substandard pharmaceuticals. The difference is that they are deliberately and fraudulently mislabeled with respect to identity and/or source. These products mostly have no therapeutic benefit; they can cause drug resistance and death" (WHO, 2006). Brand names that have been counterfeited include Viagra, Lipitor, Zyprexa, Ambien, Xanax, Lexapro, Ativan, Tamiflu, and others. Generic versions of these drugs are also frequently counterfeited and often contain heavy metals, including aluminum and uranium, which gradually kill the patients, often via cardiac arrhythmias. In other cases, death is instantaneous, as the superpotent narcotic fentanyl is often substituted for alprazolam, zolpidem, and other controlled drugs. One of the most counterfeited drugs in the world is Viagra. An internet search to purchase Viagra online yields millions of results, many of which claim to offer the cheapest Viagra prescriptions online, and even

Viagra without a prescription! Most of these websites advertising Viagra and other prescription medications are unregulated and fraudulent. In fact, it has been estimated that 95 percent of internet pharmacies are bogus (Partnership for Safe Medications). You are spinning the roulette wheel and betting your life when you order Viagra (and other drugs) online.

It is bad enough that careless profiteers are willing to introduce contaminated drug products into our supply chain. Imagine the magnitude of the tragedy that would arise if a rogue group of bioterrorists were to *intentionally* introduce megaquantities of intentionally subpotent or superpotent drugs. For example, we could easily have millions of people bleeding out if anticoagulants were potentiated or have people becoming hypercoagulable if the same drugs were rendered subpotent.

In fact, it's already happening:

The danger associated with an insecure supply chain was highlighted in January 2008, when FDA responded to a crisis involving the contamination of the active pharmaceutical ingredient (API) used to manufacture heparin, a potent injectable anticoagulant used to prevent and treat blood clots. The contaminated heparin, which was associated with numerous adverse events—including deaths—came from a facility in China. During its investigation, FDA determined that some manufacturers were not adequately safeguarding their heparin supply chains. The heparin supply chain starts with a raw source material, primarily derived from the intestines of pigs, that is processed into crude heparin. Thousands of small pig farms in the Chinese villages extract and process pig intestines in small workshops called casing facilities. Consolidators collect different batches of heparin from various workshops and sell these batches to manufacturers, who further refine the crude heparin into heparin API, the active ingredient used in heparin drug products and heparin containing devices. More than half of the finished heparin products in the United States and globally are made from Chinese-sourced materials. (GAO, 2011)

FDA officials identified statutory changes that the organization believed it needed to help improve its oversight of drugs manufactured in foreign establishments. For example, in place of the current requirement that FDA inspect domestic establishments every two years, officials indicated the agency would benefit from a risk-based inspection process with flexibility to determine the frequency with which both foreign and domestic establishments would be inspected. In light of the growing dependence on drugs manufactured abroad and the potential for harm, FDA needs to act quickly to implement changes across a range of activities in order to better assure the safety and availability of drugs for the US market (GAO, 2011).

https://www.reuters.com/article/us-china-pharmaceuticals/
special-report-chinas-wild-east-drug-store-idUSBRE87R0OD20120828

Until recently, FDA did not have field offices overseas. In 2008 FDA finally opened its first office in China:

Established in November 2008, the China Office serves as the lead for FDA's on-site presence in China. The mission of the Beijing-based office is to help ensure the safety, quality, and effectiveness of medical products and food produced in China for export to the United States. It was important to have a local presence in China after the public health crises caused by the economic adulteration of two Chinese-produced products—pet food laced with the plastic substance melamine to cheaply boost the appearance of protein content, and contaminated heparin, the blood thinner, that had been contaminated with a related, but less expensive, chemical (GAO, 2011).

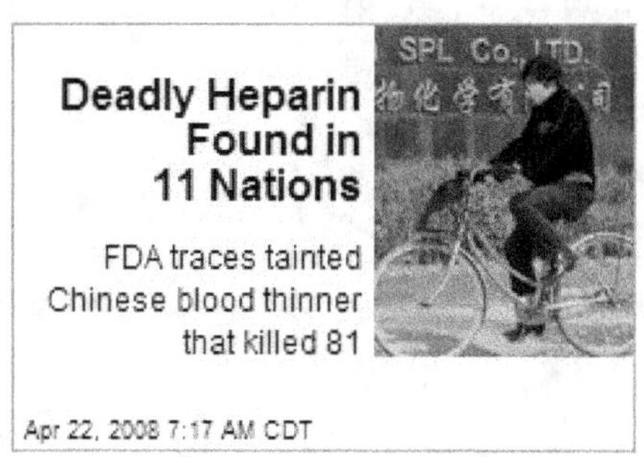

Upon investigation, FDA concluded that the heparin adulteration with a cheaper toxic synthetic alternative was an intentional cost-cutting measure to dilute the active drug product and make more money for the firm. As the owners profited, hundreds of US citizens became sick in their hospital beds with symptoms such as nausea, vomiting, excessive sweating, and rapidly falling blood pressure. In some cases, life-threatening shock occurred. In all, over one hundred US hospital patients died in their beds because of a predatory group of unregulated individuals half a world away.

https://en.wikipedia.org/wiki/2008_Chinese_heparin_adulteration

Had FDA been granted the global authority to conduct *unannounced* overseas inspections and assays, perhaps this tragedy would have been avoided. But FDA was only permitted to show up for an inspection if specifically invited. The *Wall Street Journal* stated the following: "The Chinese government didn't pursue an investigation into deadly heparin sent to the U.S. in 2007 and 2008, despite repeated requests from the U.S. for help, according to a congressional probe. Two House Republicans said Food and Drug Administration officials recently told them that the agency has been 'severely hampered' by the lack of cooperation from China in finding those responsible. Contamination in the widely used blood-thinner was linked to at least 81 deaths in the U.S." (Mundy, 2010).

In her testimony before the Committee on Health, Education, Labor and Pensions for the US Senate (GAO-11-936T), Marcia Crosse addressed this very issue as follows: "Globalization has placed increasing demands on FDA, which is responsible for the oversight of drugs marketed in the United States, regardless of whether they are manufactured in foreign or domestic establishments." While Americans once used drugs that were mostly manufactured domestically, this is no longer the case. According to FDA, the number of drug products manufactured at foreign establishments has more than doubled since 2002, with China and India accounting for the greatest share of this growth (GAO-11-936T). The 2019 GAO report (GAO-20-262T) revealed that from 2012 through 2016 the number of foreign-drug-manufacturing-establishments inspections increased. Yet the number of foreign- and domestic-drug-establishment inspections decreased by about 10 percent and 13 percent, respectively, between 2016 and 2018. FDA officials attributed the decline, in part, to vacancies among investigators available to conduct inspections. Investigators play a vital role in FDA's oversight of foreign establishments. The GAO acknowledged that FDA may have *never* inspected many foreign drug establishments manufacturing drugs for the US market. One can only imagine the plethora of good manufacturing process violations that are occurring at overseas pharmaceutical firms that have never been visited by FDA. Perhaps rats and mice are frolicking in a urine puddle as the nonbioequivalent tablets and capsules roll off the presses. Meanwhile, swarms of flies and mosquitoes circle above, playfully dive-bombing their rodent comrades. Anyone who is familiar with *The Jungle*, by Upton Sinclair, and the works of Samuel Hopkins Adams knows what happens when foods and drugs go uninspected by governmental authorities. When the cat's away, the mice will play.

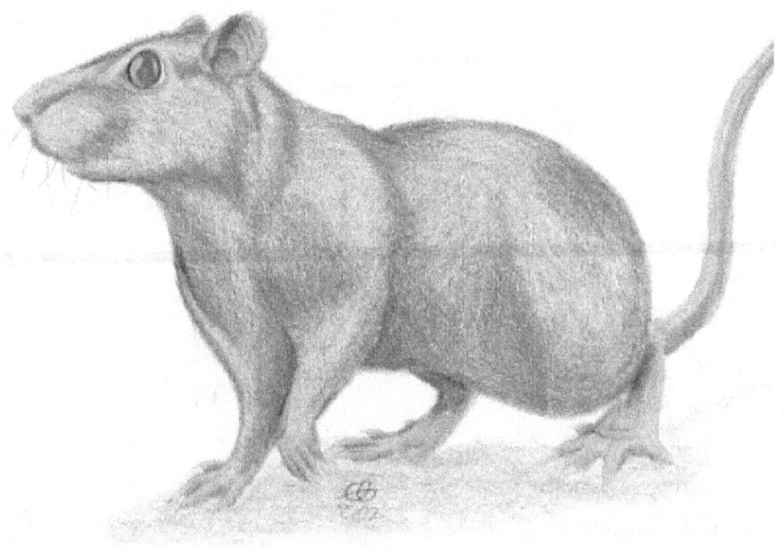

While FDA is doing its best with the resources it has available, the take-home message is clear: the medications we are taking to save us are possibly doing more harm than good because the 1938 Food, Drug and Cosmetic Act is being circumvented by China and other foreign profiteers. This travesty is not the fault of FDA, but it is unequivocally a bipartisan failure as the government neglects our national security, allowing us to devolve back to the unregulated days of the patent medicine era.

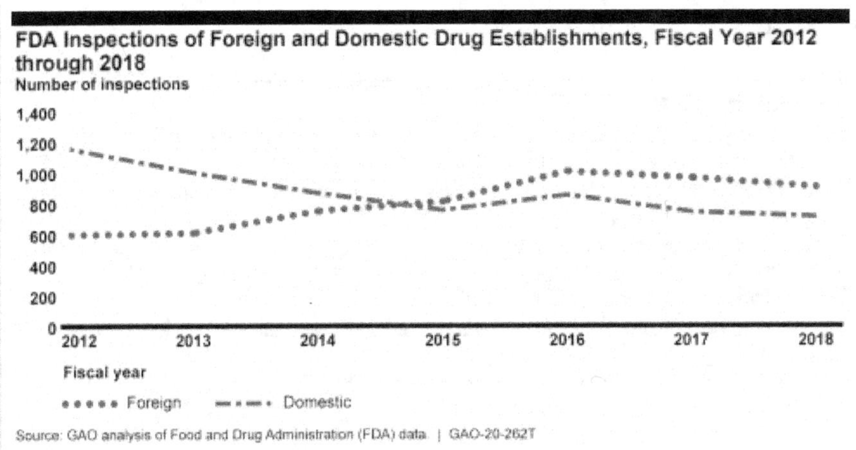

Source: GAO analysis of Food and Drug Administration (FDA) data. | GAO-20-262T

The GAO has stated, "In recent years we have reported on several aspects of FDA's ability to protect Americans from unsafe and ineffective drugs entering our supply chain. Amid growing concerns with the increasing demands placed on the agency, including its ability to ensure the quality of drugs manufactured overseas, we added FDA's oversight of medical products to our High-Risk Series. FDA has acknowledged that globalization has fundamentally changed the environment for regulating pharmaceutical products and the agency has begun taking steps to address some of these concerns, such as the establishment of overseas offices" (GAO-11-936T). The December 2019 GAO report shows that not much has changed when it comes to the challenges of conducting FDA inspections on foreign soil. FDA identified deficiencies during the majority of foreign inspections. From 2012 to 2018, FDA identified deficiencies in 64 percent of foreign-drug-manufacturing-establishment inspections. These included major deficiencies necessitating a classification of "voluntary action indicated" (VAI) and the more serious "official action indicated" (NAI).

At the time of publication, COVID-19 is still killing hundreds daily in the United States, while China, the source of the virus, is reopening. With much of the United States still under quarantine, it seems unlikely that FDA staff (through no fault of their own) will be able to travel globally to police pharmaceutical quality assurance in China, India, or anywhere else for a while. Yet uninspected nonbioequivalent drugs continue to arrive in the United States because we literally cannot live without them.

Inspection Classifications

Based on their inspection findings, FDA investigators make an initial recommendation regarding the classification of each inspection:

- **No action indicated (NAI)** means that insignificant or no deficiencies were identified during the inspection.
- **Voluntary action indicated (VAI)** means that deficiencies were identified during the inspection, but the agency is not prepared to take regulatory action, so any corrective actions are left to the establishment to take voluntarily.
- **Official action indicated (OAI)** means that serious deficiencies were found that warrant regulatory action.

Source: GAO. | GAO-20-262T

Valsartan is an antihypertensive drug used to treat high blood pressure. It can also lower the risk of death after a heart attack. In a very contemporary case from July of 2018, there was a global recall and market withdrawal of all pharmaceutical products containing the drug valsartan, which was contaminated with a known carcinogen in raw materials originating from a Chinese supplier. N-nitrosodimethylamine (NDMA) is a known carcinogen and was detected in the product manufactured by Zhejiang Huahai Pharmaceuticals Co. Ltd. Valsartan is a "maintenance" drug, meaning that most patients take this medication every single day of their lives to control their blood pressure. This indicates that the many thousands of people who have taken their medication daily as prescribed have been ingesting toxic NDMA for many years. Unacceptably, our prescription drugs, particularly the nonbioequivalent generic versions from China and India, are killing us.

This book is absolutely not about criticizing legitimate drug manufacturers that produce their products on US soil, where FDA has the regulatory power of *unannounced* inspections. We should all be very thankful to the pharmaceutical industry for extending our life spans and enhancing our quality of life. Specifically, we owe a debt of gratitude to the brand-name and generic pharma companies that help protect our national security by conducting their manufacturing here in the United States. These manufacturers generally follow all good manufacturing practices and operate in full compliance with the Food, Drug, and Cosmetic Act. We should also be grateful to FDA for its role in overseeing all the stages of drug development, drug approval, and postmarketing surveillance. Furthermore, to repeat, we must not underestimate the protective power of unannounced FDA inspections.

FDA Keeps Us Out of Harm's Way

When it comes to Americans purchasing and ingesting food and medication, FDA is the watchdog agency whose job it is to protect us from adulterated and misbranded foods and pharmaceuticals that might place us in harm's way. FDA, basing its knowledge on decades of devastating adverse experiences, knows that nothing is more important to our personal safety and our national security. Even so, millions of financially desperate American consumers continue to purchase potentially harmful drug products from outside the approved and protected supply chain. Additionally, there are numerous nefarious profiteers (individuals, corporations, and nations) that continuously attempt to undermine FDA by infiltrating our supply chains with substandard products at the expense of safety.

In today's world, the globalization of the pharmaceutical arena has put the safety of our domestic drug supply chain, and consequently our national security, in jeopardy. With almost all raw materials and finished drug products originating from overseas, FDA has the resources to conduct surprisingly few inspections of foreign drug firms. Every day, Americans consume imported nonbioequivalent generic drugs that have never been inspected by FDA.

According to the GAO report on drug safety published in September of 2011, FDA is plagued by a lack of information regarding these underregulated entities. The December 2019 GAO report on drug safety identified an understaffed FDA that has been unable to keep up with the significant challenges of overseas inspections.

It is not only the individual foreign drug manufacturers that are of concern. Each step of the manufacturing process may be outsourced to a variety of foreign vendors and subcontractors, particularly in China and India, where overall sanitation and hygiene is always questionable. Adherence to good manufacturing practices is quite unlikely, especially in the current COVID-19 environment, placing the integrity of the entire global drug supply chain in jeopardy. Even the mighty FDA is no match for COVID-19. The global spread of coronavirus has forced FDA to halt overseas pharma inspections. Virtually none of the critical pharmaceuticals—including aspirin, ibuprofen and penicillin—that we depend upon arriving from China, India, or other faraway lands are being inspected by FDA due to COVID-19.

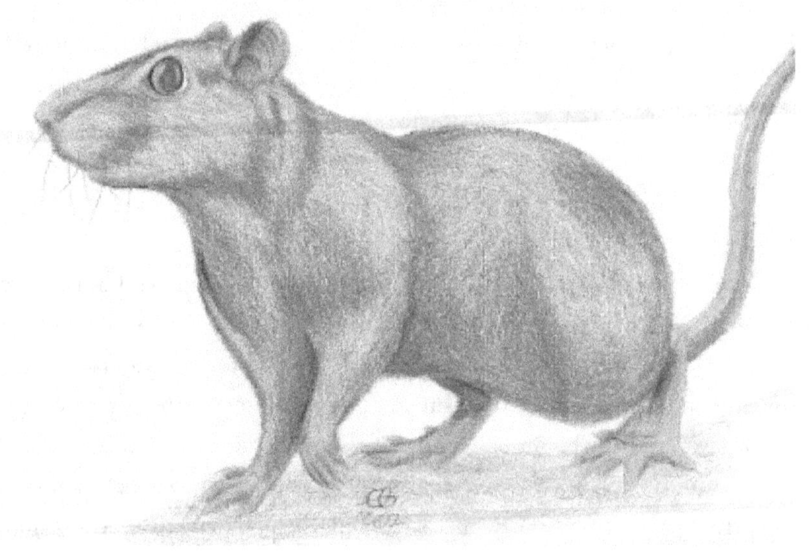

"There is no FDA, so I can play."

The critical drug shortages brought about by COVID-19 also highlight the importance of the Drug Supply Chain Security Act (DSCSA). The DSCSA's <u>Title I "Drug Compounding"</u> section provides provisions for pharmaceutical product identifications requiring manufacturers and repackagers to include unique product identifiers on prescription drug packages, including electronic bar codes. This electronic system provides the tracking of each pharmaceutical product as it moves along the supply chain, from manufacturers to wholesalers, distributors, and every other entity that has handled each product. The DSCSA mandates product verification to establish systems and processes that are able to verify the product identifier on prescription drug packages. Any drug identified as suspected of being counterfeit, unapproved, or potentially dangerous is to be quarantined and investigated. FDA must be notified if a drug is determined to be illegitimate. Theoretically, the system will enhance FDA's ability to help protect the public from *domestic* breaches in the drug supply chain. Meanwhile, the global supply chain is not a closed system, and with manufacturing occurring over seven thousand miles away, who really knows what fetid extras are getting dumped into the mixing bowls at unscrupulous Chinese drug companies? No one really knows what filth is going into our foreign-sourced drugs, and no one will ever know because there are not nearly enough FDA personnel to police the world. *The only way to protect the American public from "death by prescription" is to bring the generic pharmaceutical manufacturing industry back home.*

Although detection and removal of potentially dangerous drugs from the supply chain will better protect US patients, greedy individuals will still do their best to circumvent authority. Today, adulterated and misbranded drugs continue to find their way into the global supply chain, and everyone must remain vigilant. Sprinkled among the legitimate suppliers and distributors will always be the guy in his bathtub with an oar exporting his homemade concoctions to unsuspecting consumers worldwide. Lamentably, this incredibly intelligent counterfeiting bathtub guy also has a scanner and a high-quality laser printer. Consequently, his deadly counterfeit drugs, complete with perfectly scanned images of real pharmaceutical labels, easily slip into the global supply chain and into *your* medicine cabinet.

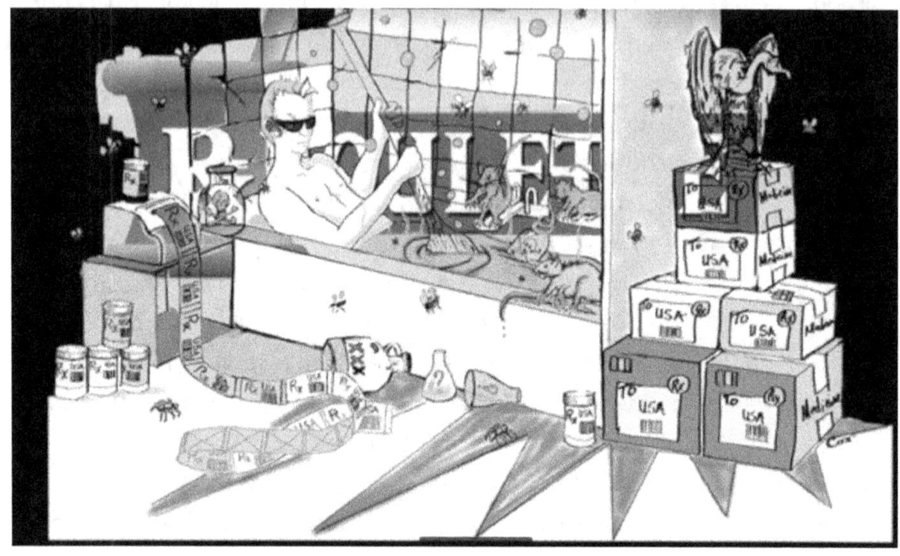

Guy in his bathtub with an oar, mixing your drugs (artist: Shelly J. Cox)

As global and domestic timelines show, the drugs we take and the foods we eat were not always as safe as they are today. For this, we need to be grateful to Upton Sinclair, Samuel Hopkins Adams, and FDA. Still, in every generation there are those individuals, corporations, and even nations that will try to rise up against us and annihilate us by slipping inferior products into our nation's drug supply chain. Recent examples include FDA's ban on naughty Ranbaxy Laboratories from distributing raw materials in the United States after finding "*flies too numerous to count*" (my emphasis) at an overseas factory (McClain, 2014; Virk, 2014). "The presence of flies in sample storage rooms and nonadherence to sample-analysis procedure were among the lapses found in Ranbaxy's plant in Punjab, India that led to the United States Food and Drug Administration banning imports made at the facility" (McClain, 2014). Here's a link to a *Wall Street Journal* article on the same subject:

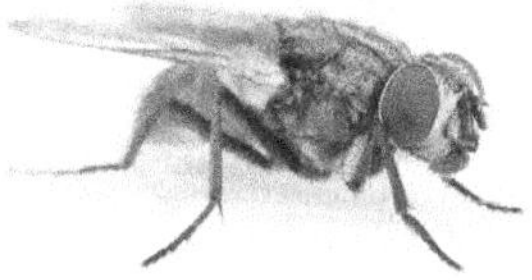

https://www.wsj.com/articles/fda-says-ranbaxy-workers-fudged-test-results-1390834130

How many years was this atrocity of an oversight going on before FDA discovered it? How many millions of doses of putrid Ranbaxy medication were consumed by our families? How many millions of doses of nonbioequivalent Ranbaxy products did unsuspecting pharmacists dispense to naive patients before the ban by FDA? Here is a link to a *New York Times* article on this critical issue:

https://www.nytimes.com/2014/02/15/world/asia/medicines-made-in-india-set-off-safety-worries.html

We as consumers, patients, caregivers, and concerned citizens must be ever vigilant of quality and safety issues pertaining to the foods and drugs we consume, especially those that may arrive in the United States from ambiguous overseas sources.

News & Events

FDA NEWS RELEASE

FOR IMMEDIATE RELEASE
September 16, 2008

Media Inquiries:
Rita Chappelle, 240-753-860
Christopher Kelly, 240-753-8
Consumer Inquiries:
888-INFO-FDA

FDA Issues Warning Letters to Ranbaxy Laboratories Ltd., and an Import Alert for Drugs from Two Ranbaxy Pl
Actions affect over 30 different generic drugs; cites serious manufacturing deficiencies

The Food and Drug Administration (FDA) today issued two Warning Letters to Ranbaxy Laboratories Ltd., of the Republic of India, and an Import Ale Ranbaxy's Dewas and Paonta Sahib plants in India.

The Warning Letters identify the agency's concerns about deviations from U.S. current Good Manufacturing Practice (cGMP) requirements at Ranba Dewas and Paonta Sahib (including the Batamandi unit), in India. Because of the extent and nature of the violations, FDA today issued an Import Ali may detain at the U.S. border, any active pharmaceutical ingredients (API) (the primary therapeutic component of a finished drug product) and both drug products manufactured at these Ranbaxy facilities and offered for import into the United States.

Clean Water

Clean water is a scarcity in many areas of the world, including the places in which many of the pharmaceuticals we consume are manufactured. Open defecation is a common practice due to lack of plumbing. Malaria, cholera, and dysentery, although rare in the United States, remain common threats in many parts of Africa and Asia. Cholera and dysentery are directly associated with fecal contamination of the water supply. This is potentially the same water used by overseas pharmaceutical manufacturers as well as counterfeiters. FDA has already received many reports of bacterial contamination of Chinese-manufactured drugs, so this is not a theoretical concern; it is a reality. Below is a transcript of warning letter sent by FDA to Zhejiang Hisun Pharmaceutical Company in China, citing deviations from FDA GMPs:

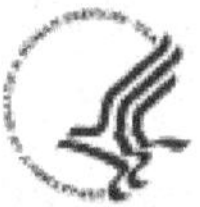

Department of Health and Human Services

Public Health Service
Food and Drug Administration
Silver Spring, MD 20993

Warning Letter: 320-16-06

Via UPS

December 31, 2015

Mr. Hua Bai, CEO
Zhejiang Hisun Pharmaceutical Co., Ltd.
46 Waisha Road
Jiaojiang District
Taizhou City, Zhejiang Province
China 318000

Dear Mr. Bai:

From March 2–7, 2015, investigators from the U.S. Food and Drug Administration (FDA) inspected your drug manufacturing facility, Zhejiang Hisun Pharmaceutical Co., Ltd., 46 Waisha Road, Jiaojiang District, Taizhou City, Zhejiang Province.

We identified significant deviations from current good manufacturing practice (CGMP) for the manufacture of active pharmaceutical ingredients (API).

These deviations cause your drugs to be adulterated within the meaning of Section 501(a)(2)(B) of the Federal Food, Drug, and Cosmetic Act (FD&C Act), 21 U.S.C. 351(a)(2)(B), in that the methods used in, or the facilities or controls used for, their manufacture, processing, packing, or holding do not conform to, or are not operated or administered in conformity with, CGMP.

We have reviewed your March 27, 2015 response in detail and acknowledge receipt of subsequent responses.

Our investigators observed specific deviations during the inspection, including, but not limited to, the following.

1. Failure to prevent unauthorized access or changes to data, and to provide adequate controls to prevent manipulation and omission of data.

During the inspection, FDA investigators discovered a lack of basic laboratory controls to prevent changes to your firm's electronically stored data and paper records. Your firm relied on incomplete records to evaluate the quality of your drugs and to determine whether your drugs conformed with established specifications and standards.

Our investigators found that your firm routinely re-tested samples without justification and deleted analytical data. We observed systemic data manipulation across your facility, including actions taken by multiple analysts, on multiple pieces of testing equipment, and for multiple drugs. You are responsible for determining the causes of these deviations, for preventing recurrence, and for preventing other deviations from CGMP.

a. During the inspection, we reviewed the electronic log for high performance liquid chromatography (HPLC) system #36 and determined that the audit trail was disabled on February 6, 2014. One of your analysts executed 80 HPLC injections for assay and impurity tests of validation stability batches **(b)(4)** of **(b)(4)** API.

Because the audit trail was disabled, neither your quality unit nor your laboratory staff could demonstrate that records for these batches included complete and unaltered data. All supporting raw data was discarded, including sample solution dilutions and balance weight printouts. Sample analyses were not recorded in the instrument use logbook. Test results were deleted from the hard drive and all supporting chromatograms were discarded. Audit trail functions were re-enabled on February 8, 2014, and the same analyses were repeated. You submitted the February 8th test results to FDA in March 2014 in support of Drug Master File (DMF) **(b)(4)**.

During the inspection, we asked the analyst who generated the data submitted to FDA whether audit trails could be disabled. The analyst stated that another employee, who was no longer with the company, had disabled the audit trails. Your firm could not explain why the audit trail was disabled or why the original data was deleted, nor could you demonstrate whether the original results were within specification.

In your response, you assumed that the original raw data was deleted because a system suitability failure invalidated the data. You acknowledged that the data should not have been invalidated without an investigation of the laboratory event. However, your response is inadequate. There is no evidence to support invalidation of the original data on the grounds of a system suitability failure because your firm deleted all of the original records associated with these analyses.

b. While reviewing the electronic log for HPLC system #28, we determined that two of your analysts deleted portions of HPLC sample sequence 20140221 during assay, impurities, and identity testing for **(b)(4)** API batches **(b)(4)**, and **(b)(4)**.

During the inspection, the investigator reviewed the data package that your firm used for batch release decisions for this drug. This data package included results from 44 HPLC injections. However, the electronic audit trail from the instrument used to generate these results showed that there were a total of 61 injections. Raw data for 17 of the 61 injections was deleted from the reported sequence as if the injections had never been performed. The investigator later discovered the missing data in a backup folder.

You stated in your response that these specific API batches "were sold to [the] Chinese market" and that you planned to retest batches **(b)(4)** to determine whether they are within specification.

You also stated in your response that the missing portions of the sample sequence were actually injections conducted for training, so product quality was not affected by the deletions. This response is inadequate, because, regardless of the reason for conducting the injections, your laboratory records must retain all original raw data.

c. While reviewing the audit trail on HPLC system #28, we determined that one of your analysts performed trial HPLC injections during assay and impurities testing for batches of **(b)(4)** API (**(b)(4)** and **(b)(4)**). These trial injections were performed on May 4–6, 2014. The data for the sample set was deleted from the system. Testing was not recorded in the instrument use logbook. All supporting electronic raw data was discarded. Testing results for these batches were then recorded on May 7, 2014, when the analyses were repeated using HPLC system #32.

During our inspection, one of your analysts provided the original analyses worksheets to review. According to this analyst, tests were repeated because of poor column efficiency. The analyst neither initiated an investigation of the laboratory event nor documented the original analyses in the instrument use logbook. The analyst did not respond when we asked why the initial chromatograms were deleted.

However, in your written response, you claimed that this analyst later recalled deleting the data (chromatogram) because column inefficiency may have invalidated the data. Your quality unit must review all pertinent analytical data when making batch release decisions. When analysts delete nonconforming test results, the quality unit is presented with incomplete and inaccurate information about the quality of the products. Your response does not demonstrate how your laboratory procedures prevent the deletion of data or how the quality unit ensures that the records relied upon for batch release and other quality review decisions are complete and accurate.

Our concerns about deletion of data are heightened by the significant number of customer complaints for subpotency and out-of-specification (OOS) impurity levels from 2012–2014. We observed data deletion in your laboratory related to assay and impurity levels during this time period. During the inspection, we asked to review your lab's raw analytical data of the lots associated with four of the 61 complaints. However, you were unable to provide the raw data because it had been deleted. Without raw test data for the lots associated with these complaints, your firm could not adequately investigate the complaints, nor could you expand your investigation to determine whether other lots were affected by the same problems or take corrective actions, such as recalling drugs if appropriate.

We acknowledge your commitment to hire a third-party consultant, set up user access restrictions, and upgrade computerized systems with audit trails. However, simply activating audit trail functions and instituting password controls are insufficient to correct the broad data manipulation and deletion problems observed at your facility and to prevent their recurrence.

Your management is responsible for the assuring that the scope and extent of the third-party audit is adequate, including a full evaluation of sophisticated electronic systems and their potential for manipulation. Your management is also responsible for fully documenting and preserving records.

For more information about handling OOS results and documentation of your investigations, please refer to *Investigating Out-of-Specification (OOS) Test Results for Pharmaceutical Production* at http://www.fda.gov/downloads/Drugs/Guidances/ucm070287.pdf and *Questions and Answers on Current Good Manufacturing Practices, Good Guidance Practices,*

Level 2 Guidance—Records and Reports at http://www.fda.gov/Drugs/
GuidanceComplianceRegulatoryInformation/Guidances/ucm124787.htm

The problem here lies within the fact that many of the incoming raw materials and finished drug products circumvent scrutiny by FDA. Through no fault of their own, workers in Africa and Asia are often forced to live and work in dangerous, dirty, and demeaning environments. As an advocate of public health, I empathize with these people. I strongly believe that we must help them by providing resources for the creation of cleaner and safer living, working, and manufacturing environments. With much of the pharmaceutical supply being sourced from areas where billions of individuals and businesses lack access to clean water, we are currently experiencing a tsunami of substandard drugs entering the US marketplace. It is entirely plausible that water used in the overseas manufacturing processes could be teeming with *E. coli* or other pathogenic organisms. Our FDA would be none the wiser from thousands of miles away and without global authority to conduct quality control tests on the water supply. With the majority of active pharmaceutical ingredients and finished drug products coming from overseas nations that have water stress and water insecurity, mainly China and India, we have very valid cause for concern. On the contrary, I know from my own working experience that every source of water in every US manufacturing facility is routinely tested to make sure it is free of pathogenic contamination.

With China controlling the majority of the world's drug supply, we are seeing a continuous flow of low-quality drug products entering the global supply chain. China does not have good manufacturing practice laws. Consequently, "anything goes" when it comes to the potential ingredients that are contained in drugs arriving from China. Whatever ingredients the proverbial roulette wheel lands on—that is what goes into the drug-mixing blenders at the generic Chinese pharmaceutical firms.

Upton Sinclair wrote *The Jungle* in 1905 to expose the dangerous and unsanitary conditions in the meatpacking industry in turn-of-the-century America. *The Jungle* was an assigned reading in my tenth-grade American history class, and I read it from cover to cover—twice. Years later, while working as a pharmacist and personally observing the tsunami of generic drug recalls, I began to realize the similarities between the frequent headlines in the *Wall Street Journal* and Sinclair's *The Jungle*. Sinclair, a muckraker, went undercover in Chicago and exposed an industry where diseased and rotten meat was routinely being released for public consumption. Atrociously, if a person were to slip and fall into the meat grinders, they simply became part of the food product. Needless to say, the public was shocked at Sinclair's revelations. The White House was inundated with mail demanding reform of the meatpacking industry. Sinclair's work was strongly supported by President Theodore Roosevelt, and the two communicated frequently, with Sinclair being invited to the White House for a meeting. As a result, President Roosevelt selected a special commission to investigate Chicago's slaughterhouses. In May 1906, the commission issued a scathing report that corroborated the atrocities that Sinclair had identified:

Passage of the Meat Inspection Act opened the way for Congress to approve a long-blocked law to regulate the sale of most other foods and drugs. For over 20 years, Harvey W. Wiley, chief chemist at the Department of Agriculture, had led a "pure food crusade." He and his "Poison Squad" had tested chemicals added to preserve foods and found many were dangerous to human health. The uproar over *The Jungle* revived Wiley's lobbying efforts in Congress for federal food and drug regulation. The same day that President Roosevelt signed the Meat Inspection Act, he also signed the Pure Food and Drug Act, regulating food additives and prohibiting misleading labeling of food and drugs. This law led to the formation of the federal Food and Drug Administration. (Constitutional Rights Foundation, 2019)

Today, FDA is the only entity that stands between putrefied foods and drugs and the American public.

In a situation similar to Upton Sinclair's *The Jungle* from one hundred years ago, if a rodent (or any creature, great or small) falls into the Chinese drug mixture today, it will simply become part of the finished drug product; no one in the factory will report it, and no one in the factory will care. The finished drug product—rodent included—will end up in your medicine cabinet and in your bloodstream. If Upton Sinclair and Samuel Hopkins Adams were alive today, I would not be writing this book because they would have already coauthored it.

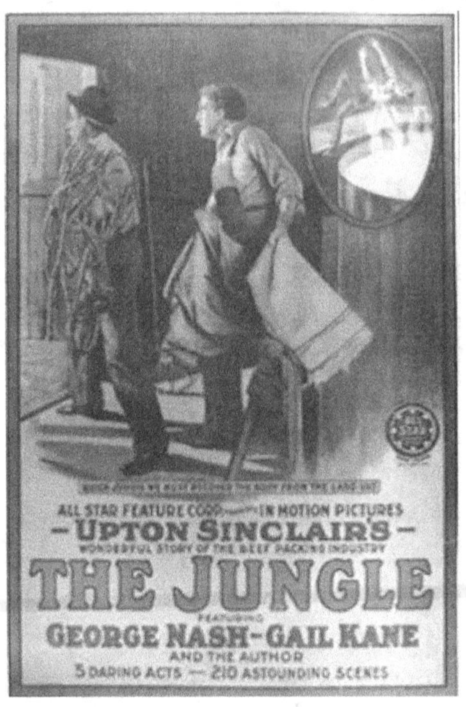

Ironically, the recent drug shortage inflicted by the coronavirus has high-lighted the global dependence on China within the world's pharmaceutical supply chain. The limited availability of potential remedies for COVID-19, as well as critical shortages of virtually all the pharmaceuticals and medical supplies that we normally depend upon, exemplifies the dangers of reliance on overseas suppliers (Gao et al., 2020; Gautret et al., 2020; Yao et al., 2020). It is unacceptable that not only do we tolerate nonbioequivalent drugs flowing in from China and India, but we also depend upon them. It is time for the United States to stop relying on inferior foreign drugs and other medical imports and regain its Big Pharma dominance for brands as well as generics. The 1938 Food, Drug, and Cosmetic Act was designed to protect us from crude and shoddy drugs. Now, we have become dependent on them. The time has arrived for the United States to again begin manufacturing and stockpiling our own generic drugs. We must revitalize our domestic generic pharmaceutical industry so that we can be better prepared for, and less dependent on, future interruptions of the unreliable global pharmaceutical supply chain. It's time to stop playing health care roulette. Additionally, this shortage also extended to the ventilators, N95 masks, and other critical medical supplies necessary to combat COVID-19. Meanwhile, many of the replacement masks being imported from China continue to fail quality assurance tests such as "the fit test," which ensures that the respirator mask is properly fitted to the individual's face type to provide the safest protection. Furthermore, instead of the superior N95 masks, inferior KN95 masks are being substituted. These do not offer the same protections to frontline health care workers who are caring for COVID-19 patients. Over 1,300 fraudulent Chinese medical suppliers have used the same fake US postal address of record for a nonexistent American agent (CCTC Service Inc.) in order to export substandard masks into the United States. Due to the critical shortage of personal protective equipment, these inferior masks made by King Year Printing and Packaging Company Ltd. (WSJ, 2020) were used in health care facilities despite having failed quality measures, putting countless US medical personnel at risk (Hufford, 2020). Additionally, counterfeit masks, intended to mimic medical-grade N95 masks made by the Shanghai Dasheng company have already infiltrated Canadian and US hospitals (cbc.ca).

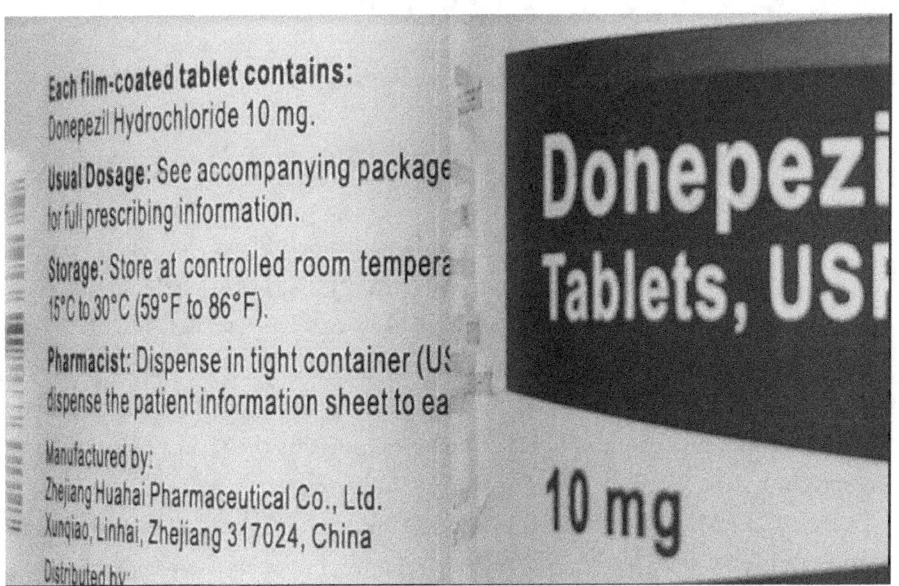

Potentially uninspected Chinese made drugs are on your pharmacists' shelves right now. Adulterated and misbranded Chinese pharmaceuticals manufactured by Huahai and others continue to flood global markets, despite countless FDA recalls.

What could be better than this example of how foreign drug importation is not the answer to our drug shortages? Have we not learned our lessons? Here is an informative link to an FDA website that discusses the importation of drugs:

https://www.fda.gov/ForIndustry/ImportProgram/ucm173751.htm

Pharmacy Benefit Managers

The first pharmacy benefit manager (PBM) was called Pharmacy Card Systems Incorporated, also known as PCS and Advanced PCS. In the early 1970s, PCS invented the plastic benefit card that most of us carry in our wallets to this day. PBMs originally acted simply as claims processors, known as third-party administrators and fiscal intermediaries, by adjudicating pharmacy prescription drug claims by paper and eventually via computers. For this they were paid a fee per prescription.

Today's PBMs have morphed into unscrupulous drug middlemen that nontransparently broker deals in pay-to-play schemes between themselves, clients, brokers, insurance companies, and pharmaceutical manufacturers. PBMs decide what drugs may be dispensed, how much they will pay for a drug, and the out-of-pocket patient co-pay. Pharmaceutical manufacturers are shaken down and forced to pay up in order to get lucrative preferred status and pole position on formularies. PBMs inflate co-pays, overcharge payers and patients, under-pay providers, and pocket the spread (difference). Excessive co-payments and coinsurances inflict direct financial burden and are intentionally used to drive patient behaviors. Many patients are forced to forego filling their prescriptions due to unaffordability.

PBMs are supposed to save the system money with the aggregate buying power of millions of enrollees via their private or government health plans. Sponsors and patients supposedly save money on their prescription drugs through price discounts, rebates from pharmaceutical manufacturers, and PBM-owned mail-order pharmacies that home-deliver prescriptions. Not only are mail-order patients deprived of their rights to face-to-face pharmacist consultations, but the PBMs also falsely tout their highly profitable mail-order service as a cost-saving measure. Watch this video, which proves otherwise:

https://www.youtube.com/watch?v=LO8agu-ftFQ

As exposed in a recent documentary, PBMs actually pocket much of the monetary savings, rather than passing it along to their clients and patients. Health care providers, insurers, and PBMs are supposed to follow the principle of benefi-cence, which means always acting in the best interest of the patient, not toward the financial gain of a middleman. PBMs specifically prevent pharmacists from sharing cost-saving information with patients because the PBMs pocket the dif-ference between the cash price and the insurance price. *By artificially inflating co-pays to bolster their own bottom lines, PBMs intentionally deter patients from filling their necessary prescriptions, thus contributing to increased morbidity and mortality* (Austvoll-Dahlgren et al., 2008; Eban, 2013; Gourzoulidis et al., 2017; Lyles et al., 2016; Pawasakar et al., 2018; Shah, 2009).

Senior citizens on fixed incomes cannot afford the inflated co-pays imposed by PBMs and are forced to choose between paying for food and filling their prescriptions. In many cases seniors are financially compelled to circumvent the safety net of FDA and seek out potentially deadly imported "Canadian" knockoffs at deeply discounted prices. These "Canadian" drugs may appear to ship from north of the border, but they are often nonbioequivalent counterfeits manufactured in some distant cesspool without FDA oversight. Counterfeit drug products continuously pour into the US drug supply chain. It is estimated that twenty illegal online pharmacy websites go live every day. In early 2020, due to contamination with NDMA, the Canadian government recalled certain brands of the medication metformin, which millions depend upon to control their type 2 diabetes.

Globalization of the pharmaceutical supply chain has placed increasing demands on FDA in ensuring the safety and effectiveness of drugs marketed in the United States, as well as those pharmaceuticals entering the supply chain illegally, thus circumventing the safety net of FDA. The influx of deadly uninspected pharmaceuticals from abroad, combined with frantic patients seeking cheaper drugs via the internet, makes for a prescription for disaster. Astronomical drug prices are a burden on many Americans' budgets. Adults who do not take prescription medications as prescribed due to unaffordable out-of-pocket expenses have been shown to have poorer health status, increased hospitalizations, and more cardiovascular events.

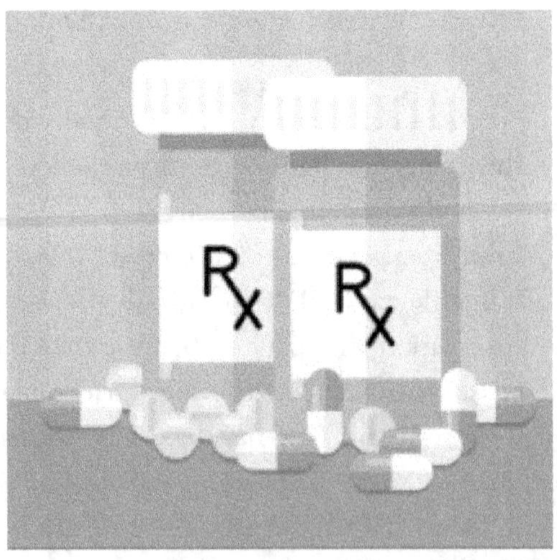

The benefits that could be derived from lower out-of-pocket costs are vast. Existing studies by Gourzoulidis et al. (2017), Shah (2009), Pawasakar et al. (2018), Lyles et al. (2016), and many others unequivocally link unaffordable pharmacy co-pays *directly* to adverse health outcomes in the form of increased morbidity (disability) and mortality (death) in persons with diabetes and other chronic diseases. These scientific studies represent *real news*, published in credible peer-reviewed journals. Rather than acknowledging the continuous rhetoric spewed by PBMs and (some) politicians, my references cite studies that provide an irrefutable connection between the medical literature and the many real-life examples of human suffering. *Nonadherence to prescribed insulin and other prescription drugs due to PBM-induced co-pay unaffordability is killing US persons every single day.* Here is the link again to the *Wall Street Journal* article explicitly blaming the PBMs for unaffordable insulin prices:

https://www.wsj.com/articles/insulin-prices-soar-while-drugmakers-share-stays-flat-1475876764

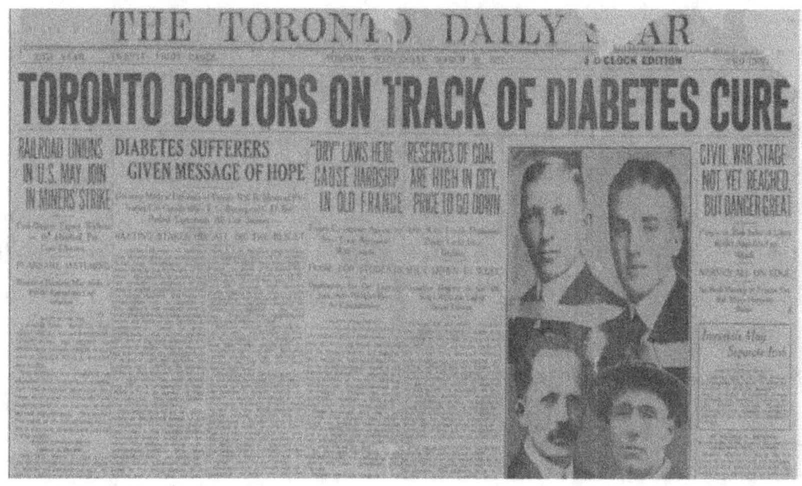

PBMs never take physical possession of actual prescription medications. Thus, they bear little to no risk, yet they reap huge kickbacks in determining which medications will appear on the formulary of each drug plan. In order to further intimidate prescribers, PBMs use restrictive prior authorizations as a weapon to keep lifesaving medications out of the reach of sick patients. Hence, even items that are supposedly "covered" on the PBM's formulary either never get approved or are accompanied by unaffordable price tags (co-pays). When insurers try to save money by shifting the cost burden to the patient, medication adherence goes down because patients can no longer afford to take their medications as prescribed (Austvoll-Dahlgren et al., 2008). It is unfathomable that in the year 2020 diabetics are being denied access to the only antidote that can save their lives, but here is the proof:

https://www.npr.org/sections/health-shots/2018/09/01/641615877/
insulins-high-cost-leads-to-lethal-rationing

Big Pharma Is Our Savior

It costs hundreds of millions of dollars for Big Pharma to bring a drug to market, and Big Pharma has a finite amount of time to recoup its research and development expenditures before "me-too" generics enter the marketplace. Manufacturers are entitled to make a profit. In fact, Big Pharma must make a profit in order to fund future research and development and keep new drugs in the pipeline. If drug companies cannot make a fair profit, research and development will be stifled. Unlike PBMs, which are only glorified claims processors, Big Pharma plays a critical role in preventing, treating, and curing sickness and disease. Hundreds of thousands of people across the world have already been wiped out by COVID-19. Without the development of tests, treatments, and vaccines, the coronavirus pandemic might easily prove more disastrous than the Spanish flu of 1918, which killed upward of one hundred million people. We did not have jet airplanes in 1918, so it took a bit longer for the Spanish flu to find its way across the globe by sea. COVID-19, within weeks, became the worst pandemic the world has experienced since 1918.

Our fate now depends on the innovation of our Big Pharma superheroes, including Gilead Sciences, Pfizer, GlaxoSmithKline, Sanofi, Regeneron, Johnson & Johnson, Amgen, and AstraZeneca, as well as biotech firms like Moderna, CytoDyn, Novavax, and Inovio. Gilead Sciences is cranking out its antiviral drug remdesivir, which was originally developed to treat hepatitis C and the Ebola virus. Remdesivir was recently granted emergency authorization by FDA to treat coronavirus patients. Moderna and Inovio are conducting clinical trials on vaccines. One fact is certain: you are never going to see an insurance company or a PBM invest their dollars to save the world from a pandemic. Meanwhile, China and others are attempting to sabotage our innovative efforts by stealing our research data (Sanger, 2020). Not only is this industrial espionage; it is a direct assault on our public health and our national security.

Research and development by universities and Big Pharma aimed at bringing a vaccine to market are the only things that might save us from the multiple waves of COVID-19 that scientists guarantee will take place as the United States and the world reopen in order to avoid complete and permanent economic collapse. As the final edits are being completed for the second printing of this book on Memorial Day, 2020, thousands are flocking to the beaches. One of the problems with COVID-19 is that infected people who are subclinical (not clinically ill) are still capable of spreading the virus (Gordis, 2014). Infections without obvious signs of clinical illness are still important because we do not really know for sure if we are face-to-face with an infected person—or even whether we are infected ourselves. This is why social distancing and wearing a mask is recommended by the CDC. According to the *Wall Street Journal*, "China, Singapore, South Korea, Iran and Germany are among a handful of countries that have seen signs of the virus re-emerging as stringent containment measures have been relaxed" (Ansari, 2020). Additionally, there is no guarantee that those who have recovered from COVID-19 have immunity to a second infection.

We often complain about high drug prices, taking for granted lifesaving advances such as immunizations, antibiotics, and insulin. Yet, if not for Big Pharma, type 1 diabetes would still be a death sentence, as it was prior to the discovery of insulin in 1921 by Drs. Banting and Best, and Eli Lilly's bringing insulin into the marketplace in 1922. Thankfully, today we have Eli Lilly, Novo Nordisk, and Sanofi cranking out the lifeblood for patients with diabetes. If not for Big Pharma, we would not have insulin or any new drugs for multiple myeloma and other cancers—and we would all be doomed from COVID-19. *Thank you to all of the insulin manufacturers for keeping the supply chains open during the COVID-19 pandemic and keeping diabetes patients alive. Thank you to all of the innovators who are working on therapies to treat, cure, and prevent COVID-19.*

Compared with the United States, drug prices are significantly less expensive in many overseas countries. In Europe governments directly or indirectly control drug costs. In the United States, insurers, PBMs, and hospitals negotiate drug prices. In Europe the government dictates the price that manufacturers must adhere to if they want to do business. Yet, if we were to impose government price controls on medications, we would remove the incentive behind the research and development of lifesaving new drugs that are now allowing people to achieve normal life spans while living with or being cured of diseases (cancer and HIV/AIDS, for example) that were considered untreatable until recently. Scientists spend many years studying for a reason. We must allow free market pricing in the drug industry if we want developers to continue to search for cures. Otherwise we will continue to devolve to the days when millions died of mass pandemics for which there were no cures. COVID-19 is proving the value and dedication of Big Pharma to the health and well-being of the American people and the world at large. *Let us never take the research and development of our branded pharmaceutical industry for granted.* Big Pharma is investing its own capital, ingenuity, and technology in the fight against the coronavirus. Let us never permit noninnovators to introduce nonbioequivalent generics into our supply chain. Let us always prevent PBM drug middlemen that care more about the price of their stock than the health of their participants from driving up drug prices and shifting the costs to patients.

Let us not forget the peer-reviewed references cited in this book that clearly explain the direct connection between not being able to take one's medication due to cost and the increase in morbidity and mortality. The research is unequivocal: PBMs are decreasing the quality and quantity of the American life span. Perhaps it is not too late to follow the lead of West Virginia, which in 2017 cut out the for-profit drug middlemen from its Medicaid managed-care program. According to Bloomberg, "By running the program itself and eliminating spreads and reducing administrative fees, it expects to save $30 million a year—about 4 percent of the state Medicaid drug spending" (Langreth, 2018). Bravo to West Virginia, but these bold actions need to be taken at the federal level, not one state at a time.

https://www.bloomberg.com/graphics/2018-drug-spread-pricing/

The corner drugstore, best exemplified by Jimmy Stewart in Frank Capra's 1945 movie *It's a Wonderful Life*, will soon be gone if the general public and lawmakers do not take the steps necessary to preserve this pillar of the community. Small drugstores are thorns in the sides of PBMs, just as George Bailey was a thorn in the side of greedy Mr. Potter in Capra's film. Just ask any independent pharmacist how many times he or she has *personally* dropped off medicine to a sick patient late at night or on a Sunday afternoon. In these times of COVID-19, independent pharmacies are on the front lines serving their patients, like they have for over one hundred years. While independent pharmacies used to deliver 10 percent of their prescriptions, due to COVID-19 they are now delivering (free of charge as they always have) 90 percent of their prescriptions. Here is a link to an interview that includes a discussion regarding PBM transparency and disclosure. Click on this link, or paste it into your web browser:

https://www.youtube.com/watch?v=Swdz4fisicQ&feature=youtu.be.

Private insurance companies, Medicare, and even cities like the town of Rockford, Illinois, hire PBMs to do negotiating for them. Recently, CBS News accurately exposed a PBM as an evil villain, having multiple potential conflicts of interests by not only owning a PBM but also owning a mail-order pharmacy that profits each and every time a prescription is filled.

Simultaneously, the big three PBMs financially strong-arm patients into using mail-order services rather than patronizing their community pharmacies. By offering three months' supplies via the mail for lower co-pays than community pharmacies are permitted to charge, PBMs ignore the "any willing provider" rules and illegally steer the patients directly into their own respective mail-order or brick-and-mortar pharmacies. While they may save the consumer a co-pay, they are billing the payers (employers) prices that are eight to ten times higher than those available in retail settings.

The only entities *benefiting* in these self-referral schemes are the PBMs—perhaps that's how they got their middle name. Patients, physicians, employers, and pharmaceutical companies are all victims of this unregulated industry. PBMs are double-dipping as the claims processor *and* the provider pharmacy, *paying themselves fees and making money in all directions*. Last but not least, the PBM auditors circle back to local mom-and-pop pharmacies again, months later, like sharks, to finish off their prey in the form of recoupment of hundreds and thousands of dollars for minor clerical errors or, often, for no legitimate reason whatsoever. Meanwhile, who audits the PBMs' own mail-order pharmacies? Here is a link to a great interview with a pharmacist with over thirty years of experience serving the community. He gives a spectacular account of how PBMs are intentionally causing the demise of the institution of community pharmacy. Scan the QR code here, or paste the URL into your web browser:

https://www.youtube.com/watch?v=Swdz4fisicQ&feature=youtu.be.

In the near future, you, the patient, will depend solely upon PBM-owned mail-order delivery of lifesaving prescription drugs. These drugs may be exposed to extreme temperatures, causing the drugs to melt in the summer and freeze in the winter. The drug insulin, for example, is a fragile protein and the perfect example of a drug that must be kept refrigerated within a certain temperature range. Extreme heat or cold will easily denature the protein, rendering the insulin useless. Type 1 diabetes patients will quickly develop diabetic ketoacidosis and die without their insulin. Type 2 diabetes patients may present with hyperosmolar nonketotic syndrome, which manifests as potentially fatal hyperglycemia (ADA, 2020). Would *you* want to risk *your* life using insulin that was potentially exposed to extremes in temperature, sitting in cold warehouses, traveling on sweltering hot delivery trucks, or waiting on your doorstep in the middle of August or February? Or how about having your medications dropped down the chimney on Christmas Eve via a PBM drone? During the COVID-19 pandemic, it has been local community pharmacies, not mail-order warehouses, that have been personally helping patients get their medications immediately upon request. If patients wish to utilize mail-order drug delivery, they should absolutely be permitted to do so. However, this is America, and mail-order should be an option—not a mandate.

https://www.pbs.org/newshour/show/
do-prescription-drug-middlemen-help-keep-prices-high

Our health care system is a sloppy and complex maze, consisting of a hodge-podge of governmental payers such as Medicare and Medicaid, private (for-profit) insurance companies, and individuals paying out of their own pockets. Large out-of-pocket expenses in the form of premiums, deductibles, co-pays, and non-covered goods and services often deter people from seeking medical treatment in the earliest stages of illness, when many conditions are easily curable. Delaying seeing a provider can prove detrimental or even deadly. Often these high out-of-pocket expenses are designed to discourage usage of the insurance coverage!

Many PBMs contractually prohibit pharmacists from telling patients that the cash price for a prescription may, in many cases, be cheaper than running the claim through the insurance company. Here is this very important link to auditor general Eugene DePasquale reminding consumers how to save money by circumventing the PBM robber barons:

https://www.youtube.com/watch?v=h2_yDTU5kJw&feature=youtu.be

One size does not fit all when it comes to prescription drug dosing. The elderly, by definition, have compromised kidney and liver function. It takes them longer to metabolize and clear drugs from the body. In order to avoid the accumulation of drugs in the body, the elderly generally require lower doses or wider intervals between doses. Too high a dose or too many doses spaced too close together, and the drugs begin to accumulate, making the patient susceptible to increased side effects. In an elderly patient, a broken hip means months in a rehabilitation facility, reduced quality of life, and even an earlier-than-anticipated trip to the cemetery. But if a potential error is noticed, the pharmacist can reach out to the prescriber to double-check the order.

These services are all provided for free and are just part of the everyday responsibilities of community pharmacies that go unrecognized and unacknowledged. Meanwhile, the conveyor belts of the PBM-owned mail-order behemoths keep moving, and the emphasis is placed on speed and volume. Through no fault of their own, chain and mail-order pharmacists are pressured to keep the orders flowing, not unlike the Domino's Pizza business model, except with much more dire consequences when an error is made. Again, it's not the pharmacist's fault, but the chain behemoths and PBMs want those prescriptions filled lickety-split, just like any other commodity! The National Academy of Medicine estimates that every year, approximately 1.5 million patients are harmed by preventable pharmacy medication errors. Hospitals spend $3.5 billion extra as a result of preventable medication errors annually (Nationalacademies.org). Speed, all too often, comes at the expense of accuracy. Always check the description and appearance of your medications to make sure that your prescriptions have been filled accurately before you take them. Unfortunately, you may still have no way of knowing if they are nonbioequivalent Chinese knockoffs that have never been inspected by FDA.

A Google search of PBMs will immediately bring up a treasure trove of relevant, controversial articles regarding PBMs and their clandestine practices. Here is a link to an unbiased CBS video interview with a PBM; you can come to your own conclusions:

https://www.youtube.com/watch?v=LwosYxSkTAM.

PBMs had more of a secretarial role in the 1970s in the United States. They were simply claims processors. Today PBMs are multibillion-dollar enterprises that generate revenue for themselves on the false premise that they decrease prescription drug costs. PBMs steer patients to their own networks of preferred pharmacies (which they often own), including mail-order pharmacies, thus maximizing their revenue while jeopardizing patient safety and denying patients the freedom to choose their own providers. PBMs are not innovators and do not invest in research and development. They work to earn revenue for their stockholders via high out-of-pocket prices to patients, secret backdoor kickbacks extorted from manufacturers, pay-to-play schemes forced upon manufacturers, and unfair charge-backs and audits at the pharmacy level. These kickbacks exist at all levels, including Medicaid, Medicare, and commercial sectors. Instead of backdoor rebates to middlemen, there should be transparent upfront discounts to patients at the pharmacy counter. Meanwhile, automatic shipping keeps your drugs coming whether you need them or not, generating huge profits for the mail-order firms and PBMs while generating a huge waste of accumulated unused drugs.

Each PBM has a preferred chain pharmacy that it works with, mandating that its members use that chain rather than an independent pharmacy. In some cases, the chain drugstore, insurance company, and the PBM are under one corporate umbrella, collecting fees, rebates, and co-pays from all directions simultaneously. A recent Bloomberg article gave an example in which a large PBM was managing the drug benefit plan for a jail in Iowa and had billed the county for $198.22 for one bottle of generic antipsychotic pills. The contracted dispensing independent pharmacy was paid only $5.73 for the services it provided, including filling and delivering the prescription. The other $192.49 went directly to the bottom line of the PBM, as the county got overcharged and the pharmacy got paid less than its cost to provide the services. Now, Wapello County Jail bypasses the PBM middleman and purchases its pharmaceuticals directly from the independent pharmacy that actually renders the products and services (Langreth, 2018).

National Public Radio has produced an excellent clip of describing how PBMs pocket the lion's share of the revenue:

https://www.npr.org/sections/health-shots/2017/08/02/540918790/
video-little-known-middlemen-save-money-on-medicines-but-maybe-not-for-you

Mergers between insurance companies and PBMs create antitrust violations and represent a major conflict of interest not only when it comes to small pharmacies being excluded as providers but also in decreasing the freedom of choice that patients have regarding the right to choose their own providers of pharmaceutical services. Mail-order drug pharmacies create a mammoth amount of waste by automatically shipping unnecessary medications, as I have previously discussed.

https://www.youtube.com/watch?v=LO8agu-ftFQ

To be sure, these patients will be receiving their prescriptions from the mail carrier, with no pharmacist interaction except via telephone or internet, a thousand miles away. This is acceptable if that is what each individual patient prefers. The choice should be left up to each individual patient to select the pharmacy that he or she wishes to patronize. Every time the Department of Justice gives the green light to these types of vertical health care mergers, it creates a major conflict of interest; this is an injustice to consumers who have patronized local corner drugstores for generations. Countless community pharmacies have been forced to close their doors due to relentless cuts in reimbursements by PBMs. With patients forced to use a particular chain pharmacy or mail-order dispensary, these providers will now have a captive audience (you) that can be made to wait forever to receive their lifesaving medications via mail or drone. Fewer pharmacists and technicians will be needed on staff at these drug giants because the patients will (contractually) not have the option of going to another pharmacy, thus being forced to wait as long as it takes. The vertical mergers between insurers, PBMs, and chain pharmacies facilitate deceptive antitrust practices that bring in millions of dollars in revenue to these newly formed monopolies. Explore the following link to read more on this topic:

http://wallerlawblog.com/post/591/cigna-express-scripts-cvs-aetna-deals-continue-vertical-integration-in-health care/

Insured patients using branded products including insulin and many inhalers for COPD and asthma are forced to pay out the wazoo. It has become commonplace for US citizens to circumvent the PBMs and drive to Canada, where insulin can be purchased (without insurance) for a fraction of the cost. Additionally, although the generics are cheaper alternatives to their brand-name counterparts, PBMs still pad the costs of many prescriptions by eight to ten dollars. Generic drugs are so inexpensive relative to branded drugs that PBMs can easily add ten dollars to every prescription when billing their clients, and no one questions it. This is known as "spread pricing" and goes straight to the bottom line of the PBM, adding up to astronomical profits. The big three PBMs are included in the top twenty-five Fortune 500 companies (*Fortune*, 2013). In many cases, patients can actually save money by paying cash directly at the pharmacy counter or with the help of a service called GoodRx. By searching for a prescription drug, GoodRx will share prices and coupon discounts across national pharmacies (GoodRx.com).

Insurance companies and PBMs have one thing in common with casinos—the house always wins. We undoubtedly have an uphill battle in our game of health care roulette because PBMs assess outcomes in terms of satisfying their stockholders rather than giving a hoot about the health and wellness of their most important stakeholders—the patients. In a traditional game of casino roulette, the player wagers on a particular number or color, winning or losing a finite amount of money. In health care roulette, the stakes are higher. You are forced to bet your life on whether you can afford your drug co-pay or whether you have to go without filling your prescription. Additionally, there is no guarantee as to whether the prescription in your bottle is real or counterfeit, subpotent or superpotent, benign, therapeutic, or instantly deadly. One day soon, China will decide to replace all of their active pharmaceutical ingredients with placebo (or something worse) so that it can conquer the world. We must reclaim our generic drug industry before it's too late.

GLOSSARY OF TERMS

accountable care organizations. Groups of physicians, hospitals, and
other health care providers and suppliers who work in tandem to administer high-quality health care while reducing costs.

active drug ingredient. The actual drug that exerts the pharmacological
effect. For example, acetaminophen is the active ingredient in the drug
Tylenol.

adulteration. A legal term meaning a food or drug that fails to meet federal
or state standards. Adulteration usually refers to noncompliance with
health or safety standards as determined, in the United States, by the Food
and Drug Administration (FDA) and the US Department of Agriculture
(USDA). Adulterated products include illegally imported fake drugs concocted in unknown conditions thousands of miles away, perhaps by a guy
in his bathtub with an oar. This is the risk you take if you purchase your
drugs from the internet.

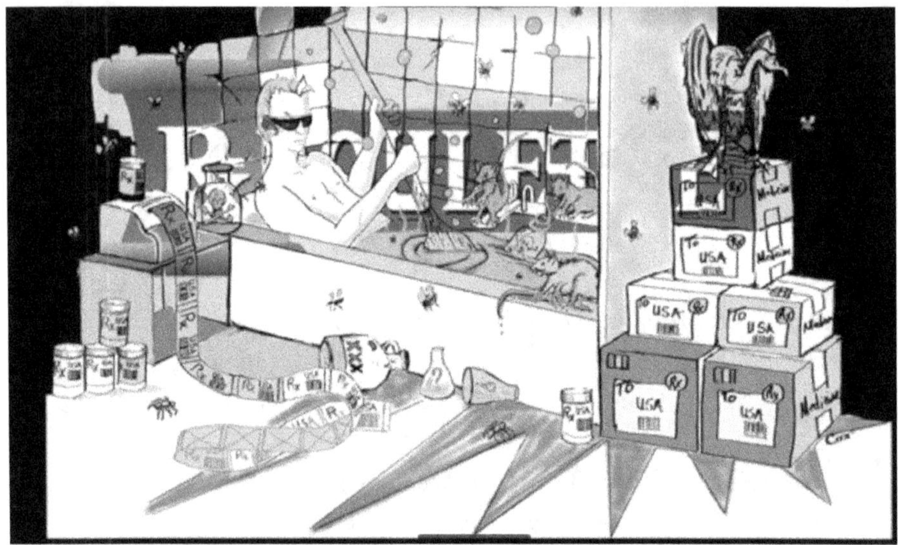

Guy in his bathtub with an oar, mixing your drugs (artist: Shelly J. Cox)

adverse drug event. Injury resulting from medical intervention related to a drug, including medication errors, allergic reactions, and drug overdosages. Adverse drug events account for hundreds of thousands of hospital admissions every year. Follow this link to read about the government's plan to prevent adverse drug events:

https://health.gov/hcq/pdfs/ade-action-plan-508c.pdf

Affordable Care Act. Also known as "Obamacare," this law is intended to promote health insurance at affordable rates, expanding the ranks of the insured and their levels of coverage, thus reducing the costs of health care.

You can read the Affordable Care Act in its entirety, at your leisure, by visiting the following link:

https://www.health care.gov/where-can-i-read-the-affordable-care-act/.

antitrust laws. Laws designed to encourage market-driven competition, providing more choices for consumers of health care. Unfortunately, the continued vertical mergers between large insurers, chain pharmacies, and pharmacy benefit managers are circumventing the antitrust laws and taking away consumer choices.

beta cells. Located within the pancreas, these specialized cells are in control of making insulin. In persons with diabetes, the beta cells are either destroyed by an autoimmune process (type 1) or incapacitated to some degree (type 2).

beneficence. Health care providers, insurers, and PBMs are supposed to follow the principle of beneficence, which means always acting in the best interest of the patient, not toward the financial gain of a middleman. This principle is ignored by PBM robber barons.

Big Pharma. *Big Pharma* is an umbrella term encompassing all the major pharmaceutical manufacturers that spend billions of dollars on research and development of new lifesaving treatments and cures. Big Pharma is often blamed for high drug prices. But without the research and development funded by drug companies, we would not have insulin to treat diabetes, antivirals to treat and cure HIV/AIDS, inhalers to save the lives of asthma patients, vaccines to prevent disease, antibiotics to cure disease, and chemotherapy to extend the lives of cancer patients. *Without Big Pharma, we would have zero chance of treating, curing, and preventing COVID-19.* The culprits behind criminally high drug costs in the United States are pharmacy benefit managers, not Big Pharma. Other countries do not have pharmacy benefit managers, and neither should the United States.

caregivers. The unsung heroes who actually spend the most amount of time with the elderly and special-needs individuals. They are often the hardest-working members of the team and deserve more recognition for the important services they provide to our loved ones. Certified nurse assistants (CNAs) and direct support professionals (DSPs) are two of the titles often associated with those who provide direct care.

carfentanil. An animal tranquilizer used in darts to bring down large mammals, including elks and elephants. It has much higher opioid activity than fentanyl. The toxicity of carfentanil has been compared to that of nerve gas.

CDC (Centers for Disease Control and Prevention). A first-responder-based agency that focuses on conditions here at home. The CDC's primary mission is to protect health and promote quality of life through prevention and control of disease, injury, and disability. The CDC has a comprehensive website that focuses on a wide array of preventative measures for those in America and those who plan to travel. The CDC focuses on (1) healthy people in healthy places, (2) preparing citizens for emerging health threats, (3) positive international health, and (4) healthy people at all stages of their lives.

co-payment. The out-of-pocket cost that a patient has to pony up at the doctor's office or pharmacy counter. Often, a patient can get drugs for less money than their co-pay simply by asking the pharmacist, "What is the cash price?" Watch this video clip right now for some very useful information regarding co-payments:

https://www.youtube.com/watch?v=h2_yDTU5kJw&feature=youtu.be

counterfeit. Fake drugs that are, by definition, adulterated and misbranded. Counterfeit drugs are often contaminated with potentially deadly impurities that may include virtually anything. The correct active ingredient may be present in subpotent (not enough) quantity or in superpotent (too much) quantity. The drug could contain zero active ingredients (refer to the Avastin example in this book). The drug could be laced with the deadly opioid fentanyl or the superdeadly opioid carfentanil, which is one hundred times more potent than fentanyl and kills instantly. Counterfeit drugs may enter the supply chain through repackagers, importers, and internet pharmacies.

deductible. The out-of-pocket expense that patients are required to pay before their health benefits start to pick up the payments.

determinants of health. The range of personal, social, economic, and environmental factors that influence our health status—biological and genetic makeup, individual behaviors, social interactions, the built environment, and access to health care.

diabetes. Diabetes is a chronic, debilitating disease that occurs when the pancreas becomes incapable of producing adequate amounts of the hormone insulin and/or when the body cannot effectively take up and utilize the insulin that is produced. Diabetes is classified as either type 1 or type 2, depending on the above criteria. Diabetes is an epidemic afflicting thirty million people in the United States and a pandemic with five hundred million people affected worldwide (WHO, 2019). Diabetes is currently classified as the seventh-leading cause of death in the United States. Diabetes is the leading cause of blindness, kidney disease, and lower-extremity amputation and is a major contributor to heart disease and strokes.

dose-limiting toxicities (DLTs). Unacceptable side effects that would force the treatment to stop (or continue at a reduced dose). The term *unacceptable* is relative; severe nausea and vomiting would probably be considered unacceptable (and therefore DLTs) for a headache remedy but not for a chemotherapy drug. It's all about benefit versus risk, and for each drug a group of experts decides what reactions constitute a DLT.

doughnut hole. A coverage gap in Medicare Part D that starts after the beneficiary and the insurer have spent a predetermined amount for the covered drugs.

Drug Supply Chain Security Act (DSCSA). Also Title II of the Drug Quality and Security Act enacted in November 2013; this law promises to transform the way the US drug supply chain operates by replacing a patchwork of pedigree requirements with an enhanced product-tracing solution for prescription drugs. It also raises licensure standards throughout the United States. The product-tracing requirements, assisted by FDA guidance, will be gradually implemented over a ten-year period.

drugs. Include, among other things, articles intended for use in the diagnosis, cure, mitigation, treatment, or prevention of disease, as well as components of those articles.

effectiveness. How well the treatment works in the real world, where people might refuse to take it as directed (or at all) because of its unpleasantness and/or its side effects.

efficacy. How well a treatment works in an ideal situation in which every patient takes his or her medication exactly as prescribed.

epidemic. Disease spreading rapidly across a large number of people, in excess of what is normally to be expected in a defined community, geographical area, or season.

epidemiology. Study of disease incidence, prevalence, and distribution patterns among populations. Epidemiology is the foundation of public health because its focus is to prevent disease from occurring and reoccurring.

excipients. Inactive ingredients that accompany active drug products, included as "filling agents," "bulking agents," "stabilizing agents," or "flavoring agents." These supposedly "inert" substances serve as vehicles or media for pharmaceutical delivery. Excipients represent a very vulnerable component of the drug supply chain. Counterfeiters and unscrupulous overseas manufacturers can easily slip adulterated products into the drug supply chain by providing cheaper excipients to save money or to cause intentional harm to patients. US citizens (as well as the entire world) should be vigilant in inspecting the sources of the medications they take because instead of extending your life, they may abruptly end your life.

facilitators. Storefront pseudopharmacies that masquerade as Canadian drugstores in US strip malls. Not licensed pharmacies at all, these middlemen accept prescriptions from the general public, often senior citizens who cannot afford their co-pays. The prescriptions are mailed off, supposedly to Canadian pharmacies, and the patient receives a mail-order shipment of drugs to his or her front door. The individual ingredients that make up these drugs are sourced from all corners of the world, especially China, where pharmaceutical regulation is still in the Stone Age. There has been an exponential increase in drug recalls due to contaminants discovered in Chinese (and other foreign) drug products easily crossing our borders and finding their ways into *your* medicine cabinets. Yes, you—the reader—are personally at risk of this breach of FDA's safety net. *If you are a senior citizen* *and you want to remain alive to see your grandchildren grow up, please heed this warning and do not purchase your medications from the internet.* Explore the following link to see what happens when you purchase drugs from Canada:

https://www.abcactionnews.com/money/consumer/taking-action-for-you/
popular-online-canadian-pharmacy-ordered-to-shutdown-over-counterfeit-medicine

Federal Food, Drug, and Cosmetic Act of 1938. Set of laws passed by Congress in 1938 giving authority to the US Food and Drug Administration (FDA) to oversee the safety of food, drugs, and cosmetics.

fentanyl. An opioid pain medication that is often mixed with heroin or cocaine. It has a rapid onset and is used by injection, through patches applied to the skin, nasally, or by mouth. Fentanyl and its superpotent form, carfentanil, contribute to many fatal opioid overdoses in the community, as heroin users are not aware of the presence of these deadly additives. In 2016 more than twenty thousand deaths occurred due to overdoses of fentanyl and fentanyl analogues, accounting for half of all opioid deaths. It's likely that most of the victims had no idea that their heroin had been cut with fentanyl or the superpotent carfentanil.

food desert. Geographic areas that do not offer access to affordable healthy foods, including fruits, vegetables, low-fat milk, poultry, fish, and whole grains. Residing in a food desert is correlated with less healthy diets and higher incidence of diabetes and other chronic diseases, particularly for those individuals without access to vehicles.

gag clause. Restriction in pharmacy benefit managers' contracts that prohibit pharmacists from disclosing vital information to a customer that would reduce his or her out-of-pocket expenses for medications. Many inexpensive generic pharmaceuticals would be much cheaper for patients to simply pay for out of pocket, bypassing the insurance. PBMs steer uninformed patients to have all the claims go via the insurance, artificially inflating the co-pays. The "spread" is pocketed by the nontransparent PBMs. If you have not yet viewed this video, please view it now to save money on your prescriptions:

https://www.youtube.com/watch?v=h2_yDTU5kJw&feature=youtu.be

generic drug. A pharmaceutical that is considered equivalent to the innovator (brand) drug but that no longer has patent protection. This allows multiple manufacturers to begin producing the product, thus lowering the price through competition. Although generic drugs such as metformin and others may cost only pennies to produce, PBMs often exploit the consumer by artificially inflating co-pays as well as astronomically overcharging the employer or health plan, pocketing the spread.

health disparities. Health disparities refer to differences in access to health care services as well as to the quality of the care that people actually receive. There is a higher incidence and prevalence of sickness, injury, morbidity, and mortality experienced by certain populations. Health disparities are typically correlated with the social determinants of health. For example, those of lower socioeconomic status and less education have poorer outcomes compared to those who have higher incomes, more education, and social capital.

health promotion. Public-health-related educational, social, and environmental interventions designed to encourage healthy behavior among the overall population as opposed to focusing on individuals.

herd immunity. Resistance to the spread of a contagious disease among those who are susceptible because enough people are immune that transmissions have slowed or stopped.

incidence. The number of new cases of a particular disease within a population in a given time period.

insulin. A hormone that facilitates the entry of glucose from the bloodstream into the cells, where it is needed for energy. The best analogy to comprehend this concept is to envision insulin as the key that unlocks the cells so that glucose can enter. Insulin was discovered in 1921 by Drs. Fredrick Banting and Charles Best, who gave the patent away to the world for free. Today, we are in the midst of the worst diabetes epidemic known to mankind. Thanks to greedy PBMs, diabetic patients cannot afford their astronomical pharmacy co-pays for insulin. Patients with diabetes are often forced to forego their lifesaving insulin therapy because PBMs will not even allow compassionate pharmacists to financially assist patients who cannot afford their co-pays. Follow this link or type it into your browser to see how people are suffering and dying because they cannot afford to purchase their lifesaving insulin:

https://www.cnn.com/2019/03/04/health/insulin-price-humalog-generic-eli-lilly-bn/index.html

intervention. Action taken to improve a particular condition or situation. For example, public health professionals often intervene in order to help promote change in the determinants of health. Intervention includes providing information, policies, and programs to produce specific health outcomes. Goals of interventions include reduction in diseases and their risk factors.

life expectancy rate. The average years that a person in any particular country is expected to live. Life expectancy is based on measurement of mortality rates from each age group in a population in a particular year. This information provides a summary of the average number of years of life remaining for those of a particular age. It implies the number of years of expected life at birth.

Misbranding. A drug is misbranded if its label is false or misleading. Counterfeit drugs, for example, may contain contaminants or impurities that are not noted on the label. Additionally, perhaps the active ingredient is not present in the quantity represented on the label. In the Avastin example noted in this book, there was no active ingredient present at all, and the cancer patients basically received placebos rather than the chemotherapy that may have otherwise saved their lives.

https://www.abcactionnews.com/money/consumer/taking-action-for-you/
popular-online-canadian-pharmacy-ordered-to-shutdown-over-counterfeit-medicine

moral hazard. The predisposition for those who have health insurance to use it for its full value and benefit. As more covered health care services are utilized, health care spending will rise proportionally or even astronomically. Moral hazard raises costs, and insurers defend themselves against it by implementing cost-sharing measures such as premiums, deductibles, and co-pays.

Narcan (naloxone). An opioid overdose can be reversed with the drug naloxone. This reversal is only temporary, and the caregiver must call 911 or the patient will relapse and die. This is because the duration of action of the opiate is longer than the duration of action of the Narcan. Naloxone is a medication that rapidly, but temporarily, reverses an opioid overdose.

The National Institutes of Health (NIH). With headquarters in Bethesda, Maryland, a research-based agency that works toward researching, preventing, and curing disease globally. The NIH is the primary federal agency for research toward prevention and control of disease worldwide. The NIH operates as part of the US Department of Health and Human Services and is the nation's medical research agency. The NIH was instrumental in the discovery that fluoride prevents tooth decay and that lithium is useful in bipolar disorder. It introduced vaccines for hepatitis, *Haemophilus influenzae*, and human papillomavirus.

opioid. Opioids are a class of drugs that includes the illegal drug heroin, synthetic opioids such as fentanyl, and pain relievers that are filled legally by prescription such as oxycodone, hydrocodone, codeine, morphine, and many others. The opioid epidemic claims over one hundred lives per day in the United States. All opioids are chemically related and interact with opioid receptors on nerve cells in the body and brain. Opioid pain relievers produce euphoria in addition to pain relief and can therefore be abused when taken more frequently or in higher quantities than prescribed. Even when prescribed by a doctor, opioid usage frequently leads to dependence, addiction, overdose, and death. *Everyone in the community, especially those who have loved ones using opioids, should have access to Narcan and be trained in the use of Narcan to save the life of a loved one who is using opioids.* Do not wait! Ask your doctor and pharmacist now about getting Narcan to keep on hand for opioid overdose emergencies. You can save a life!

pandemic. Epidemic of a global magnitude. While an epidemic might affect one nation or geographic area, a pandemic might span many nations and multiple continents. Examples of pandemics include the Spanish flu of 1918, as well as the current COVID-19 pandemic. The diabetes pandemic is proving to be a complicating comorbid contributor toward poor COVID-19 outcomes.

pharmacodynamics. The study of what the drug does to the body.

pharmacokinetics. The study of what the body does to the drug.

pharmacy benefit manager (PBM). Third-party middlemen that are hired by entities such as Medicare, Medicaid, and other governmental and private insurers to provide and manage prescription drug benefits for their members. PBMs are contractually obligated to save money for their sponsors and plan members.

https://www.npr.org/sections/health-shots/2017/08/02/540918790/
video-little-known-middlemen-save-money-on-medicines-but-maybe-not-for-you

prevalence. The number of individuals within a population who have a particular disease at a given time. Prevalence is a "snapshot" in time and is typically measured as a percentage.

primary prevention. Focuses on reducing the development of sickness and disease. Smoking-prevention and smoking-cessation programs, for example, can help reduce the occurrence of many diseases, including cancer, emphysema, and chronic bronchitis. Primary prevention emphasizes education and can prevent the disease or condition before it sets in by focusing on behaviors such as getting all recommended immunizations, adopting a healthy lifestyle including diet and exercise, and undertaking other proactive measures. The diabetes epidemic is a great example of how lifestyle modifications can reduce risk.

public health. Aims to prevent disease, decrease morbidity and mortality, increase quality of life, and promote physical health and well-being through organized community efforts for a clean and healthy environment, control of community-acquired diseases, and the education of individuals and populations regarding personal hygiene to maintain a standard of living for health maintenance.

secondary prevention. Secondary prevention, using diabetes as our example, can help those with prediabetes (the medicalized term for "borderline" or "a touch of the sugar") from progressing to diabetes (Conrad, 2007).

social determinants of health. Disparities exist in access to health care, as defined by the social determinants of health, which include race, ethnicity, socioeconomic status, age, sex, disability status, sexual orientation, gender identify, stress, housing, unemployment, and residential location right down to the zip code. Disadvantaged individuals are often marginalized or discriminated against and will ultimately incur increased complications, higher treatment costs, and more frequent hospitalizations. If you have not already viewed this video, please watch it now:

https://www.pbs.org/video/scetv-specials-zipcode-your-neighborhood-your-health-full-program/

spread pricing. The monetary difference between what PBMs charge employers, health plans, and government payers and their actual cost of doing business. Additionally, patient co-pays are inflated, and pharmacy reimbursements are grossly and unfairly reduced to the point of unprofitability. All this money is pocketed by the PBMs, going straight to their bottom lines and increasing health care expenditures. The following link, which can also be found within the text of this book, contains very useful information on how PBMs use spread pricing and inflated co-pays to drive up costs and inflate their profits. Scan this QR code, click on the hyperlink, or copy and paste it into your browser:

https://www.youtube.com/watch?v=_4_WNFPnmO8&feature=youtu.be.

tertiary prevention. Tertiary prevention can help persons already diagnosed with diabetes (for example) avoid microvascular complications (retinopathy, nephropathy, and neuropathy) that lead to blindness, ESRD, and amputations as well as macrovascular complications (heart disease, circulatory problems) (Davidson, 1981).

vector. Organism that transmits infection by conveying the pathogen from one host to another. An example of a vector is the Anopheles mosquito, which picks up the parasite plasmodium from the blood of an infected host and transfers it among others. The resulting medical condition is known as malaria. One of the biggest challenges in combating malaria in the developing world is the high prevalence of counterfeit antimalarial drugs in areas such as Africa and Asia, where malaria is endemic (Kelesidis & Falagas, 2015).

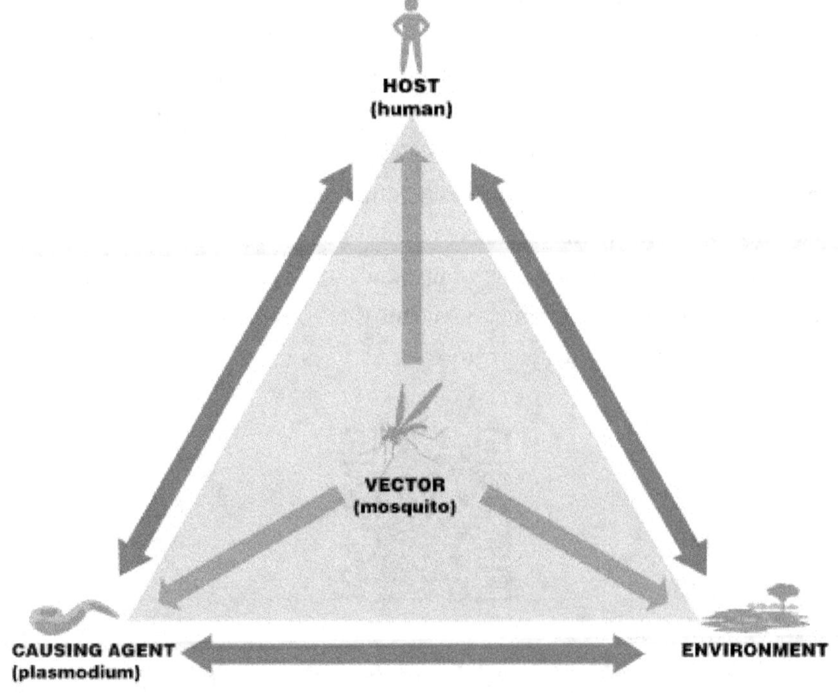

ACKNOWLEDGMENTS

I would like to express my gratitude to Mel Brodsky, who has gone above and beyond to serve and protect the profession of community pharmacy. Mel works around the clock as an advocate for the independent pharmacists in the Philadelphia region. Thank you to Elizabeth Ross for her direction in getting this book to the right people to edit and publish it in a professional and timely manner. Additionally, this book would not have been possible without the assistance provided by my friend Anthony Carfagno, who is an expert in the field of pharmaceutical regulatory affairs. Thank you to my son Jacob Tammara and my friends Dr. Adam Denish and Melissa Denish for their significant contributions to this publication. Thank you to artist Shelly J. Cox for all her work in creating the awesome cover and other artwork for this book, as well as for her contributions to my previous projects.

The majority of the statements and claims made in this book have specific references cited. Any statements made by the author that do not have references cited are the opinion of the author. The reader is encouraged *not* to rely on the opinion of the author but to draw his or her own conclusions based on real news.

ABOUT THE AUTHOR

Randolph George Tammara has been practicing pharmacy since 1992. He holds bachelor's degrees in biology and chemistry from Beaver College in Glenside, Pennsylvania. Additionally, Randolph holds a BS in pharmacy as well as a PharmD from Temple University and a master's degree in public health from Arcadia University. Having spent much of his career as a drugstore pharmacist, he now consults for long-term-care providers and acts as a certified diabetes educator. Randolph is Arcadia University's spring 2020 recipient of the Wallace E. Young Community Service Public Health Award. This award recognizes "a graduate student in Public Health or Health Education who exemplifies the spirit of community public health outreach in underserved and high-risk minority communities, and who has engaged in significant health promotion and disease prevention through direct service or education."

Randolph is passionate about combating epidemics such as obesity, diabetes, and the opioid crisis that are silently decreasing our quality of life and lowering our life expectancies. While traditional allopathic medicine focuses on treating individuals once they have already fallen ill to chronic disease, public health emphasizes a holistic approach, advocating prevention at the primary, secondary, and tertiary levels. Because less than 4 percent of health care spending goes toward prevention (Himmelstein & Woodlander, 2016), Randolph travels throughout Pennsylvania and New Jersey conducting educational in-services on diabetes and other contemporary public health issues, as well as providing long-term-care consulting services.

As a direct result of the predatory crusades by pharmacy benefit managers (PBMs) to maximize their bottom lines while specifically and deliberately causing the extinction of the traditional corner drugstore, Randolph has, reluctantly, shifted his practice away from community pharmacy. He now focuses on diabetes education, public health, and long-term-care consulting. He is a crusader against polypharmacy in vulnerable populations, including IDD and senior citizens.

Randolph's mission in *Health Care Roulette* is to provide readers with substantiated, published references and links to respected sources of information from which they can draw their own conclusions regarding who the real culprits are in the devolution of health care in the United States.

If you or your organization would like to explore the benefits of independent chart reviews for your elderly or IDD patients—or would like information regarding a PowerPoint presentation on the diabetes epidemic, pharmacology, psychopharmacology, polypharmacy, or any of the other subject matters touched upon in *Health Care Roulette*—please call Randolph Tammara toll free at 1-844-726-3364 or send an email to RanTam111@gmail.com.

AUTHOR BIOGRAPHY

Randolph George Tammara grew up working at his father's corner drugstore and observing how his father handled his customers. Tammara admired the way his father worked with them to make sure they had the lifesaving drugs they needed, whether or not they were able to pay. This generosity fueled Tammara's own career. He studied biology, chemistry, and pharmacy as an undergraduate before receiving additional pharmacy and public health degrees in graduate school.

Tammara, who lives in Philadelphia, Pennsylvania, also holds a certified diabetes educator credential. He serves his clients as a pharmacy consultant, diabetes educator, and health education trainer. For more information about his work, he invites you to visit his website, healthcareroulette.com.

REFERENCES

Adams, H. S. (1905, October 7). The great American fraud: The patent medicine evil. *Collier's Weekly.*

Ailey, S. H., Johnson, T., Fogg, L., & Friese, T. R. (2014). Hospitalizations of adults with intellectual disability in academic medical centers. *Intellectual and Developmental Disabilities, 52*(3), 187–192.

Almuzaini, T., Choonara, I., & Sammons, H. (2013). Substandard and counterfeit medicines: A systematic review of the literature. *BMJ open, 3*(8), e002923. doi:10.1136/bmjopen-2013-002923

Aleali, A., Payami, S., Latifi, S., Yazdanpanah, L., Hesam, S., & Khajeddin, N. (2018, November). Evaluation of psychological resistance to insulin treatment in type II diabetic patients. *Diabetes & Metabolic Syndrome: Clinical Research & Reviews 12*(6), 989–932.

Allen, M. (2016, May 3). Medical errors are no. 3 cause of U.S. death, researchers say. NPR.org. https://www.npr.org/sections/health-shots/2016/05/03/476636183/death-certificates-undercount-toll-of-medical-errors

American Cancer Society. (n.d.). American Cancer Society for the early detection of cancer. https://www.cancer.org/healthy/find-cancer-early/cancer-screening-guidelines/american-cancer-society-guidelines-for-the-early-detection-of-cancer.html

American Diabetes Association. (2018). Standards of medical care in diabetes. *Diabetes Care.*

Ansari, T., Yu, X., & Puko, T. (2020, May 17). As West cautiously reopens, new coronavirus infection clusters emerge in Asia. *Wall Street Journal*. https://www.wsj.com/articles/coronavirus-latest-news-05-17-2020-11589706954

Antos, J., & Capretta, J. (2018, September 16). Drug rebates aren't kickbacks. *Wall Street Journal*. https://www.wsj.com/articles/drug-rebates-arent-kickbacks-1537129846

Armental, M. (2018, July 13). FDA recalls several medicines that contain valsartan. *Morningstar*. http://news.morningstar.com/all/dow-jones/us-markets/201807139815/fda-recalls-several-medicines-that-contain-valsartan.aspx

Armour, S. (2018, October 5). Medicare splits Democrats. *The Wall Street Journal*, p. A6.

Austvoll-Dahlgren, A., Aserud, M., Vist, G., Ramsay, C., Oxman, A., Sturm, H., Kosters, J., & Verby, A. (2008, January 23). Pharmaceutical policies: Effects of cap and co-payment on rational drug use. *Cochrane Database of Systematic Reviews*. https://doi.org/10.1002/1451858.CD007017

Balick, R. (2018, June). Pharmacists stand between patients and phony drugs. *Pharmacy Today*, 31–33. https://www.pharmacytoday.org/article/S1042-0991(18)30779-5/pdf.

Barrett, D. (2015, March 30–31). UPS agrees to settle internet pharmacy case. *Wall Street Journal*, p. B3.

Bird, C., Conrad, P. Fremont, A., & Timmerman., S. (2013). *Handbook of medical sociology* (6th ed.). Vanderbilt University Press.

Bliss, M. (1982). *The discovery of insulin*. The University of Chicago Press.

Bluth, R. (2017, March 25). Welcome to Canada: Trump's promise to rein in drug prices could prompt importation laws. Kaiser Health News.

https://www.salon.com/2017/03/25/welcome-to-canada-trumps-promise-to-rein-in-drug-prices-could-prompt-importation-laws_partner/.

Bradley, E., & Taylor, L. (2013). *The American health care paradox*. Public Affairs.

Burkitt, L. (2012, April 17). China halts sale of some drugs. *The Wall Street Journal*, p. A8.

Burton, T. (2019, January 26–27). A warning on drugs for blood pressure. *The Wall Street Journal*, p. A3.

Callaway, J. (2018, July 2) Popular online Canadian pharmacy ordered to shut down over counterfeit medicine. ABC News. https://www.abcactionnews.com/money/consumer/taking-action-for-you/popular-online-canadian-pharmacy-ordered-to-shutdown-over-counterfeit-medicine

Carter, A., & Heinemann, L. (2016, October 10). If PBMs guard access to drugs, then *quis custodiet ipsos custodies?* (who will guard the guardians?). *Journal of Diabetes Science and Technology, 10*(6), 1406–1410. doi:10.1177/1932296816658056

CDC.gov. (n.d.) https://www.cdc.gov/nchs/fastats/leading-causes-of-death.htm

Cefalu, W., Dawes, D., Gaviak, G., Goldman, D., Herman, W., Van Nuys, K., Powers, A., Taylor, S., & Yatvin, A. (2018, June). Insulin access and affordability working group: conclusions and recommendations. *Diabetes Care, 41*(6), 1299–1311.

The Center for Safe Internet Pharmacies. https://safemedsonline.org/

Centers for Disease Control and Prevention. (2017). *National diabetes statistical report 2017: Estimates of diabetes and its burden in the United States*. https://www.cdc.gov/diabetes/pdfs/data/statistics/national-diabetes-statistics-report.pdf

Centers for Disease Control and Prevention (2019). National Diabetes Prevention Program (NDDP). https://www.cdc.gov/diabetes/prevention/index.html

Centers for Disease Control and Prevention. (2020, April 17). Hospitalization rates and characteristics of patients hospitalized with laboratory-confirmed coronavirus disease

2019—COVID-NET, 14 states, March 1–30, 2020. *Morbidity and Mortality Weekly,* *69*(15), 458–464. http://dx.doi.org/10.15585/mmwr.mm6915e3

Chinni, D., J. Jamerson, and D. Dougherty. (2018, September 19). Opioid crisis emerges as a dominant campaign theme. *The Wall Street Journal.* https://www.wsj.com/articles/ opioid-crisis-emerges-as-a-dominant-campaign-theme-1537349401?mod=searchresults &page=1&pos=20

Cohen, R., Kirzinger, W., & Gindi, R. (2013). Strategies used by adults to reduce their prescription drug costs. https://www.cdc.gov/nchs/products/databriefs/db119.htm

Cohn, S. Thinking of ordering discount prescriptions? Buyer beware. https://www.cnbc. com/2014/07/05/thinking-of-ordering-discount-prescriptions-buyer-beware.html https://www.congress.gov/bill/115th-congress/senate-bill/469

Conrad, P. (2007). *The medicalization of society.* The Johns Hopkins University Press.

Counterfeit Medicine. https://www.abcactionnews.com/money/. consumer/taking-action-for-you/ popular-online-canadian-pharmacy-ordered-to-shutdown-over-counterfeit-medicine

Davidson, M. (1981). *Diabetes mellitus: Diagnosis and treatment.* W. B. Saunders Company.

DEA. https://www.dea.gov/press-releases/2016/07/22/ dea-report-counterfeit-pills-fueling-us-fentanyl-and-opioid-crisis

DEA. (2016). DEA intelligence brief: Counterfeit prescription pills containing fentanyls. https://content.govdelivery.com/attachments/USDOJDEA/2016/07/22/file_attach- ments/590360/fentanyl%2Bpills%2Breport.pdf

DeNoon, D. (2008, February 28). All Baxter Heparin recalled. WebMD Health News. https://www.webmd.com/drug-medication/news/20080228/ all-baxter-heparin-recalled

DePasquale, E. (2019). Bringing transparency & accountability to drug pricing: Are rebates inflating the price of your prescription? A special report by auditor General Eugene Depasquale.

Diamond, J. (2020, May 23–24). The germs that transformed history. *The Wall Street Journal*, pp. C1–C2.

Diclemente, R., Salazar, L., & Crosby, R. (2013). *Health behavior theory for public health.* Jones & Bartlett Learning.

Eban, K. (2019, October 29). In generic drug plants in China and India, data falsification is still a problem. STAT. https://www.statnews.com/2019/10/29/data-falsification-still-problematic-china-india-drug-plants

Eban, K. (2013, October 10). Painful prescription. *Fortune.* http://fortune.com/2013/10/10/painfulprescription/

Edney, A., Berfield, S., & Yu, E. (2019, September 12). Carcinogens have infiltrated the generic drug supply in the U.S. Bloomberg.com. https://www.bloomberg.com/news/features/2019-09-12/how-carcinogen-tainted-generic-drug-valsartan-got-past-the-fda

Emanuel, E. (2014). *Reinventing American health care.* Public Affairs.

Ember, S. (2019, July 28). Bernie Sanders heads to Canada for affordable insulin. *The New York Times.* https://www.nytimes.com/2019/07/28/us/politics/bernie-sanders-prescription-drug-prices.html

Erickson, S. E., Nicaj, D., & Barron, S. (2017). Complexity of medication regimens of people with intellectual and developmental disabilities. *Journal of Intellectual & Developmental Disability.* doi:10.3109/13668250.2017.1350836

Faucon, B., Plumridge, H., & Falconi, M. (2014, May 2). Italian ring is probed in cancer-drug theft. *The Wall Street Journal*, pp. B1–B2.

FDA. https://www.fda.gov/Drugs/ResourcesForYou/Consumers/
BuyingUsingMedicineSafely/CounterfeitMedicine/default.htm

FDA. (n.d.). Looks can be deceiving: the risks of buying medicines from across the border
or around the world." Retrieved from https://www.fda.gov/drugs/resourcesforyou/
ucm078918.htm

Galewitz, P. (2016, June 6). Florida stores help consumers buy imported drugs despite federal ban. https://khn.org/news/
florida-stores-help-consumers-buy-imported-drugs-despite-federal-ban/

Galewitz, P. (2017, November 20). FDA raids Florida stores that consumers use to buy drugs from Canada. https://khn.org/news/
fda-raids-florida-stores-that-consumers-use-to-buy-drugs-from-canada/

Galvin, G. (2020, June 17). Large racial gaps in coronavirus death rates by age. *U.S. News*.
https://www.usnews.com/news/healthiest-communities/articles/2020-06-17/
stark-racial-disparities-in-covid-19-death-rates-by-age

Gao J., Tian, Z., & Yang, X. Breakthrough: Chloroquine phosphate has shown apparent efficacy in treatment of COVID-19 associated pneumonia in clinical studies. *Biosci Trends*
14(1), 72–73.

Garza, A. (2016). *Pharmacy Times Magazine*. https://www.pharmacytimes.com/publications/
issue/2016/january2016/the-aging-population-
the-increasing-effects-on-health-care

Gautret P, Lagier J, Parola P, Hoang V, Meddeb L, & Mailhe M. Hydroxychloroquine and
azithromycin as a treatment of COVID-19: Results of an open-label non-randomized
clinical trial. *International Journal of Antimicrobial Agents*. In press.

Goodman, A., Rall, T., Nies, A., & Taylor, P. (1990). *Goodman and Gilman's the pharmacological basis of therapeutics*. (8th ed.). McGraw Hill.

Goodman and Gilman's the manual of pharmacology and therapeutics. (2014). (2nd ed.). McGraw Hill.

Gokhale, K. & Narayan, A. (2014, March 7). Flies found by FDA threaten Indian town built on generics. Bloomberg.

https://www.bloomberg.com/news/articles/2014-03-06/ flies-found-by-fda-threaten-indian-town-built-on-generics

Gordis, L. (2014). *Epidemiology* (pp.13–14). Elsevier Saunders.

Gourzoulidis, G., Kourlaba, G., Stafylas, P., Giamouzis, G., Parissis, J., & Maniadakis, N. (2017, April). Association between copayment, medication adherence and outcomes in the management of patients with diabetes and heart failure. *Health Policy 121* (4), 363–377. doi:10.1016/j.healthpol.2017.02.008

Grant, Charley. (2018, August 8). Outlook darkens for drug middlemen. *The Wall Street Journal*, p. B1.

Grant, C., & Taplin, N. (2020, March 5). If coronavirus-stricken China can't export medicine, the world is in trouble. *The Wall Street Journal.*

Griffenhagen, G. https://www.pharmacist.com/sites/default/files/Great_Moments_in_ Pharmacy_Article.pdf

Harris, G. (2014, February 15). Medicines made in India set off safety worries. *New York Times.* https://www.nytimes.com/2014/02/15/world/asia/medicines-made-in-india-set-off-safety-worries.html

Hawthorne, F. (2005). *Inside FDA: The business and politics behind the drugs we take and the foods we eat.* John Wiley & Sons, Inc. https://www.health care.gov/ where-can-i-read-the-affordable-care-act/

The health care system of France [Video file]. https://www.youtube.com/
watch?v=yF69KVbUaQ www.healthypeople.gov

Hcnk, H. J., Lopes, J. M., & Bookhart, B. K. Novel type 2 diabetes medications and effect
of patient cost sharing. *Journal of Managed Care & Specialty Pharmacy, 24*(9), 847–855.
doi:10.18553/jcmp.2018.24.9.847

Hiltzik, M. (2017, June 11). How "price-cutting" middlemen are making crucial drugs vastly
more expensive. *Los Angeles Times.* https://www.latimes.com/business/hiltzik/la-fi-
hiltzik-pbm-drugs-20170611-story.html

Himmelstein, D., & Woolhandler, S. (2016). Public health's falling share of US health spending. *American Journal of Public Health.* https://ajph.aphapublications.org/doi/10.2105/
AJPH.2015.302908.

https://www.govinfo.gov/content/pkg/PLAW-113publ54/pdf/PLAW-113publ54.pdf

https://www.history.com/topics/world-war-ii/marshall-plan

https://en.wikipedia.org/wiki/2008_Chinese_heparin_adulteration

Chinese heparin adulteration. (January 2020 archived version). In *Wikipedia.* https://
en.wikipedia.org/wiki/History_of_health_care_reform_in_the_United_States#/me-
dia/File:Letter_from_Harry_S._Truman_to_Ben_Turoff_-_NARA_-_201512.tif

Holcombe, M. (2020, June 18). Florida shows signs as next coronavirus epicenter as cases
spike across the country. CNN.com. https://www.cnn.com/2020/06/18/us/us-coro-
navirus-thursday/index.html

Hopkins, J., & Roland, D (2020, February 28). FDA cites shortage of one drug, exposing supply-line worry. *The Wall Street Journal.* https://www.wsj.com/articles/
coronavirus-slows-drug-production-in-china-the-worlds-pharmacy-11582900885

Hufford, A., Maremont, M., & Lin, L. (2020, June 13–14). Over 1,300 China medical suppliers gave FDA same false U.S. address. *Wall Street Journal*, 1.

Hutt, P., & Merrill, R. (2007). *Food and drug law.* Foundation Press.

https://www.indiatoday.in/india/story/workers-skip-duty-truckers-refuse-to-move-amid-lockdown-pharma-units-warn-of-medicine-shortage-1660884-2020-03-29

Johnson, J., Stoskopf, C., & Shi, L. (2018). *Comparative health systems: A global perspective.* (2nd ed.) Jones & Bartlett Learning.

Joyce, G. (2018, August 13). Opinion: An economist's change of heart: It's time to regulate the prescription-drug middlemen. Pharmacy benefit managers find ways to boost their bottom line at the expense of employees and patients. Market Watch. https://www.marketwatch.com/story/an-economists-change-of-heart-its-time-to-regulate-the-prescription-drug-middlemen-2018-08-13?ns=prod/accounts-mw

https://www.kff.org/health-costs/press-release/poll-majorities-of-democrats-republicans-and-independents-support-actions-to-lower-drug-costs-including-allowing-americans-to-buy-drugs-from-canada/

https://kywnewsradio.radio.com/articles/news/nj-start-campaign-help-new-mothers-survive-giving-birth

Kang, H., Lobo, J. M., Kim, S., & Sohn, M. W. (2018). Cost-related medication non-adherence among U.S. adults with diabetes. *Diabetes Research and Clinical Practice, 143*, 24–33. doi:10.1016/j.diabres.2018.06.016

Kelesidis, T., & Falagas, M. E. (2015). Substandard/counterfeit antimicrobial drugs. *Clinical Microbiology Reviews, 28*(2), 443–464. doi:10.1128/CMR.00072-14

King, R. (2020, May 14). Trump administration aims to replenish strategic national stockpile to brace for 2nd COVID-19 wave. Fierce Healthcare.
https://www.fiercehealthcare.com/hospitals-health-systems/
trump-administration-aims-to-replenish-strategic-national-stockpile-to

Kripke D. F., Langer, R. D., & Kline, L. E. Hypnotics' association with mortality or cancer:
A matched cohort study. *BMJ Open, 2*, e000850. doi:10.1136/bmjopen-2012-000850

Kristof, N., & WuDunn, S. (2009). *Half the sky*. Knopf.

Langreth, D. I., & Gu, J. (2018). The secret drug pricing system middlemen use to rake in
millions. Bloomberg. https://www.bloomberg.com/grahics/2018-drug-spread-pricing.

Lee, M., & Hirschler, B. (2012, August 28). Special report: China's "wild East" drug store.
Reuters.

Lewis, K. (2009, November 10). China's counterfeit medicine trade booming. *CMAJ 181*(10),
E237–E238. doi:10.1503/cmaj.109-3070

Levitt, G. (2017, November 21). FDA actions against Canadian pharmacy storefronts in Florida. Pharmacy Checker. https://www.pharmacycheckerblog.com/
fda-pharmacy-storefronts-florida

Lizcano, K. (2016, October 25). The long and painful path of people poisoned by diethylene
glycol. Panamatoday.com.

Looney, K. (2018, October 17). Cigna-Express Scripts, CVS-Aetna deals continue
vertical integration in health care. Waller Blogs. https://www.wallerlaw.com/
news-insights/3249/Cigna-Express-Scripts-CVS-Aetna-deals-continue-vertical-
integration-in-healthcare?gs=name&gk=AETNA

Long, H. (2020, May 12). Small business used to define America's economy: the pandemic could change that forever. *The Washington*

  Post. https://www.washingtonpost.com/business/2020/05/12/
  small-business-used-define-americas-economy-pandemic-could-end-that-forever/

Lucas, A. (2020, May 7). Unproven coronavirus cures flood U.S. regulators. *Wall Street Journal.* https://www.wsj.com/articles/
  unproven-coronavirus-cures-flood-u-s-regulators-11588843805

Lyles, R, Seligman, H., Parker, M., Moffet, H, Adler, N., Schillinger, D., Piette, J., &
  Karter, A. (2015, April). Financial strain and medication adherence among diabetes
  patients in an integrated health care delivery system: The Diabetes Study of Northern
  California (DISTANCE) *Health Services Research, 51*(2), 610–624.

Maltby, E. (2012, March 22). Restocking the old machine. *The Wall Street Journal*, p. B5.

Martinez, B. (2002, August 14). Pharmacy-benefit managers at times toil for drug firms. *The
  Wall Street Journal.* https://www.wsj.com/articles/SB10292874214390016555

Maslow, A. H. (1943). A theory of human motivation. *Psychological Review, 50*, 370–396.

Mathews, A., & Chin, K. (2019, February 2–4). Cigna plays down drug-rebate overhaul. *The
  Wall Street Journal*, p. B3.

Mattioli, M., Siconolfi, M., & Cimilluca, D. (2018, November 21). Walgreens and Humana
  are in early talks to swap stakes. *The Wall Street Journal*, p. B1.

Mcclain, S. (2014, January 24). FDA says Ranbaxy workers fudged
  test results. *Wall Street Journal.* https://www.wsj.com/articles/
  fda-says-ranbaxy-workers-fudged-test-results-1390834130

McKay, B. (2018, November 18). U.S. life expectancy declines further. *The Wall Street
  Journal*, pp. A1, A6.

Moore, T. J. (1998). *Prescription for disaster.* Simon & Schuster.

Mullin, R. (2014, November 24). Cost to develop new pharmaceutical drug now exceeds 2.5B. *Scientific American*. https://www.scientificamerican.com/article/cost-to-develop-new-pharmaceutical-drug-now-exceeds-2-5b/

Nedelman, M. (2019, March 4). Amid uproar over high drug prices, Eli Lilly introduces generic insulin at half price of brand name Humalog. CNN. https://www.cnn.com/2019/03/04/health/insulin-price-humalog-generic-eli-lilly-bn/index.html

Nelson, J. (2015, November). Poor continuity of patient care increases work for hospitalist groups." *The Hospitalist*, 11. https://www.the-hospitalist.org/hospitalist/article/122016/poor-continuity-patient-care-increases-work-hospitalist-groups

Niles, N. (2018). *Basics of the U.S. health care system*. (3rd ed.). Jones and Bartlett Learning.

https://www.npr.org/sections/health-shots/2016/12/08/504667607/life-expectancy-in-u-s-drops-for-first-time-in-decades-report-finds

https://www.npr.org/sections/health-shots/2017/08/02/540918790/video-little-known-middlemen-save-money-on-medicines-but-maybe-not-for-you

O'Dwyer, M., Peklar, J., & McCallion P. (2016, June). Factors associated with polypharmacy and excessive polypharmacy in older people with intellectual disability differ from the general population: a cross-sectional observational nationwide study. *BMJ Open, 6*, e010505. doi:10.1136/bmjopen-2015-010505

OECD. https://www.oecdwatch.org/oecd-guidelines/oecd

OECD. (n.d.). United States. OECD.org. http://www.oecd.org/unitedstates/

Ozawa, S., Evans, D. R., Bessias, S., Haynie, D. G., Yemeke, T. T., Laing, S. K., & Herrington, J. E. (2018). Prevalence and estimated economic burden of substandard and falsified medicines in low- and middle-income countries: A systematic review and meta-analysis. *JAMA Network Open, 1*(4), e181662. doi:10.1001/jamanetworkopen.2018.1662

Partnership for Safe Medications. Safemedicines.org.

Patel, A. (2010, March 1). Walgreens told to pay $25.8 million over teen pharmacy tech's error. ABC News. https://abcnews.go.com/Blotter/walgreens-told-pay-285-mil-teen-pharmacy-techs/story?id=9977262

Pawasakar, M., Tang, Y., Rajpathak, G., Xu, L., Puckerein, G., & Stuart, B. (2018, October). Effect of medication copayment on adherence and discontinuation in Medicare beneficiaries with type 2 diabetes: A retrospective administrative claims database analysis. *Diabetes Therapy, 9*(5), 1979–1993.

https://www.pbs.org/newshour/show/do-prescription-drug-middlemen-help-keep-prices-high

https://www.pbs.org/video/scetv-specials-zipcode-your-neighborhood-your-health-full-program/

Peterson-Kaiser Health System Tracker. The health care system of France [Video file]. https://www.youtube.com/watch?v=_yF69KVbUaQ

Pharmaceutical Care Management Association. https://www.pcmanet.org/our-industry/

Pharmacy groups warn Trump about drug imports. (2018, June 7). *Drug Topics.*

https://pharmacy.wsu.edu/documents/2018/01/history-of-the-pharmacy-profession.pdf/

Pliny. https://en.wikipedia.org/wiki/Natural_History_(Pliny)

Przyswa, E. (2013, September). Counterfeit medicines and criminal organisations. IRACM, p. 27. https://pubchem.ncbi.nlm.nih.gov/compound/carfentanil#section=Top.

Reid, T. R. (2010). *The healing of America.* Penguin.

Reddy, S. (2018, October 9). An uphill fight against fake medication. *The Wall Street Journal*, p. A11.

Roberts, J. (2017, September 21). Big Pharma turns to blockchain to track meds. *Fortune*. http://fortune.com/2017/09/21/pharma-blockchain

Rockoff, J., & Weaver, C. (2012, April 4). FDA finds new batch of fake Avastin drug. *The Wall Street Journal*, p. B5.

Roe, S., Long, R., & King, K. (2016, December 15). Pharmacists miss half of dangerous drug combinations. *Chicago Tribune*. http://www.chicagotribune.com/news/watchdog/druginteractions/ct-drug-interactions-pharmacy-met-20161214-story.html

Roland D., & Loftus, P. (2016, October 7). Insulin prices climb, fueled by middlemen. *The Wall Street Journal*. https://www.wsj.com/articles/insulin-prices-soar-while-drugmakers-share-stays-flat-1475876764

Ruhl, J. (2008). *What they don't tell you about diabetes*. Technion Books.

Sable-Smith, B. (2018, September 1). Insulin's high cost leads to lethal rationing. NPR Weekend Edition. https://www.npr.org/sections/health-shots/2018/09/01/641615877/insulins-high-cost-leads-to-lethal-rationing

Sanger, D., & Perlroth, N. (2020, May 10). U.S. to accuse China of trying to hack vaccine data, as virus redirects cyberattacks. *New York Times*.

Scheiner, G. (2004). *Think like a pancreas*. Da Capo Press.

Schladen, M. (2019, February 19). Yost promises more actions against pharmacy benefit middlemen: "They took our money." *The Columbus Dispatch*. https://www.dispatch.com/news/20190219/yost-promises-more-action-against-pharmacy-middlemen-they-took-our-money

Schroeder, M. (2016). Death by prescription. *U.S. News* online.

Sederstrom, J. (2018, September). Prevent medication errors: Protect patients with a proactive approach. *Drug Topics*, 16–19.

Shah, N. R. (2009, February). Factors associated with first-fill adherence rates for diabetic medications: A cohort study. *Journal of General Internal Medicine, 24*(2), 233–237.

Shenolikar, R. A., Balkrishnan, R., Camacho, F. T., Whitmire, J. T., & Anderson, R. T. (2006). Comparison of medication adherence and associated health care costs after introduction of pioglitazone treatment in African Americans versus all other races in patients with type 2 diabetes mellitus: a retrospective data analysis. *Clinical Therapeutics, 28*(8), 1199–1207. https://doi.org/10.1016/j.clinthera.2006.08.012

Shenolikar, R. A., Balkrishnan, R., Camacho, F. T., Whitmire, J. T., & Anderson, R. T. (2006). Race and medication adherence in Medicaid enrollees with type-2 diabetes. *Journal of the National Medical Association, 98*(7), 1071–1077.

Slachta, A. (2018, September 5). Americans are dying because they can't afford insulin. *Cardiovascular Business.* https://www.cardiovascularbusiness.com/topics/lipids-metabolic/americans-dying-because-cant-afford-insulin

Stahl, L. (May 6, 2018). CBS News. https://www.cbsnews.com/news/the-problem-with-prescription-drug-prices/

State Health Access Data Assistance Center, University of Minnesota.

Stein, B. (2016, December 8). Life expectancy in U.S. drops for first time in decades, report finds. National Public Radio. https://www.npr.org/sections/healthshots/2016/12/08/504667607/life-Expectancy-in-u-s-drops-for-first-time-in-decades-report-finds

Stych, E. (2012, April 25). Top six UnitedHealth care group executives average $10M a year in pay. *Minneapolis/Saint Paul Business Journal.* https://www.bizjournals.com/twincities/news/2012/04/25/pay-unitedhealth-group-hemsley.html

Tadeg, H., & Berhane, Y. (2012). Substandard and counterfeit antimicrobials: Recent trends and implications to key public health interventions in developing countries.

Tam, E., & Amirfar, V. (2015). Pharmacy by vending machine. *Pharmacy Today (Journal of The American Pharmaceutical Association)*. http://www.pharmacist.com/article/pharmacy-vending-machine

Tamblyn, R., Laprise, R., Hanley, J. A., Abrahamowicz, M., Scott, S., Mayo, N., Hurley, J., Grad, R., Latimer, E., Perreault, R., McLeod, P., Huang, A., Larochelle, P., & Mallet, L. (2001). Adverse events associated with prescription drug cost-sharing among poor and elderly persons. *JAMA, 285*(4), 421–429. https://doi.org/10.1001/jama.285.4.421

Tammara, R. (2020). *The relationship between not taking medication as prescribed in the last 12 months due to cost among patients with diabetes taking insulin* (Unpublished master's thesis). Arcadia University.

Tanzi, Maria G. (2012, October). Explaining commercial interests to patients. *Pharmacy Today*, 30.

Trump, D. J. (2018, May 11). Remarks by President Trump on lowering drug prices. White House. https://www.whitehouse.gov/briefings-statements/remarks-president-trump-lowering-drug-prices/ Editorial Board

United States Government Accountability Office. (2010, September 30). *Drug safety: FDA has conducted more foreign inspections and begun to improve its information on foreign establishments, but more progress is needed* (GAO-10-961). https://www.gao.gov/new.items/d10961.pdf

United States Government Accountability Office. (2010, September 30). *The Food and Drug Administration: Overseas offices have taken steps to ensure import safety, but more long-term planning is needed* (GAO-10-960). https://www.gao.gov/products/GAO-10-960

United States Government Accountability Office (2011). *FDA faces challenges overseeing the foreign drug manufacturing supply chain* (GAO-11-936T). United States Government Accountability Office. https://www.gao.gov/products/GAO-11-936T

United States Department of Health and Human Services (2014). *National action plan for adverse drug event prevention*. United States Department of Health and Human Services. https://health.gov/hcq/pdfs/ade-action-plan-508c.pdf

United States Immigration and Customs Enforcement. (2011, January 28). Chinese national pleads guilty to trafficking counterfeit pharmaceutical weight loss drug. https://www.ice.gov/news/releases/ chinese-national-pleads-guilty-trafficking-counterfeit-pharmaceutical-weight-loss-drug

Virk, G. (2014, January 27). Ranbaxy, Daiichi Sankyo shares fall on ban. *The Wall Street Journal*. https://blogs.wsj.com/indiarealtime/2014/01/24/ ranbaxy-daiichi-sankyo-shares-fall-on-new-ban/

Weaver, C., Whalen, J, & Benoit, F. (2012, March 7). Drug distributor is tied to imports of fake Avastin. *The Wall Street Journal*, p. A14.

Wang, Jim. (2018). https://wallethacks.com/maslows-hierarchy-of-financial-needs/

Weaver, C., & Whalen, J. (2012, July 20). How fake cancer drugs entered U.S. *Wall Street Journal*, p. B4.

What the U.S. can learn about health care from other countries. (March 12, 2014). https://www.sanders.senate.gov/newsroom/recent-business/ us-can-learn-other-countries-health-care

WSJ. (2018, May 29). Why CVS loves Obamacare. *The Wall Street Journal*. https://www.wsj. com/articles/why-cvs-loves-obamacare-1527633490

World Health Organization. (2006). Counterfeit medications: The silent epidemic.

http://www.who.int/mediacentre/news/releases/2006/pr09/en/

WXPI.COM. (2019). Rising cost of insulin driving some to drive
to Canada. https://www.wpxi.com/news/top-stories/
rising-cost-of-insulin-driving-some-to-drive-to-canada/922515657

Yao X, Ye F, Zhang M, Cui C, Huang B, Niu P, Liu X, Zhao L, Dong E, Song C, Zhan S,
Lu R, Li H, Tan W, & Liu D (2020, March 9). In vitro antiviral activity and projection
of optimized dosing design of hydroxychloroquine for the treatment of Severe Acute
Respiratory Syndrome Coronavirus 2 (SARS-CoV-2). Clinical Infectious Diseases.
Advance online publication. doi:10.1093/cid/ciaa237